BIONIC PARTS FOR PEOPLE

BIONIC PARTS FOR PEOPLE

The Real Story of Artificial Organs
and Replacement Parts

by Gloria Skurzynski

illustrated by Frank Schwarz

FOUR WINDS PRESS   NEW YORK

Photo Credits

Ear Research Institute, Los Angeles, California, p. 57.
Life Magazine (Fritz Goro), p. 4.
Goodyear News Bureau, pp. 87 bottom, 120.
LDS Hospital, Salt Lake City, Utah, p. 71.
Medtronic, Inc., Minneapolis, Minnesota, p. 75.
Pennsylvania State University, p. 81 left.
Robert Regan, p. 10.
The Seeing Eye, Inc., Morristown, New Jersey, p. 18.
Roy Stevens, New York, p. 91.
Telesensory Systems, Inc., Palo Alto, California, pp. 23, 24, 25.
Texas Heart Institute, p. 81 right.
University of Utah Medical Center, pp. 12, 36, 84, 87 top,
    105, 108.
University of Wisconsin, p. 115.
Ira Wyman, p. 93

Library of Congress Cataloging in Publication Data
Skurzynski, Gloria.
    Bionic parts for people.

    SUMMARY: Discusses the invention, function, and compo-
sition of artificial kidneys, eyes, ears, hearts, arms, legs, and other
human replacement parts, and proposes some related legal and
ethical problems.
    1. Artificial organs—Juvenile literature. 2. Prosthesis—Juve-
nile literature. [1. Artificial organs. 2. Prosthesis] I. Schwarz,
Frank. II. Title.
RD130.S58   617′.95   78–54678
ISBN 0–590–07490–3

Published by Four Winds Press
A division of Scholastic Magazines, Inc., New York, N.Y.
Text copyright © 1978 by Gloria Skurzynski
Illustrations copyright © 1978 by Scholastic Magazines, Inc.
Library of Congress Catalog Card Number: 78–54678

2   3   4   5   82   81   80

For Jan

ACKNOWLEDGMENTS

The author wishes to express her gratitude to Donald Lyman, Joseph Andrade, and Stephen Jacobsen for their generous encouragement and invaluable assistance.

Special thanks are extended to Willem Kolff, Michael Mladejovsky, John Lawson, and the staff of the Division of Artificial Organs at the University of Utah; the Ear Research Institute in Los Angeles; the Cleveland Clinic; the Texas Heart Institute; the Milton S. Hershey Medical Center; Utah Services for the Visually Handicapped; The Goodyear Tire and Rubber Company; Medtronic, Inc.; Telesensory Systems, Inc.; The Seeing Eye, Inc.; to Margot Butler of the Utah School for the Deaf; to Kris Knutson, and to all the others who donated their time and efforts in the creation of this book.

CONTENTS

BIONIC PARTS FOR PEOPLE

INTRODUCTION

DURING THE PAST FEW SEASONS, TELEVISION VIEWERS HAVE watched with fascination as a fictional hero and heroine performed mighty deeds with limbs and parts made of synthetic materials. TV characters Colonel Steve Austin and Jaime Sommers hear and see, with a man-made eye and ear, far better than any human has ever heard or seen. They leap incredible heights with bionic legs and punch through walls with bionic arms. (The word "bionic" refers to machinery based on the design of living things.)

For most people, Austin and Sommers seem little more than fantasy for the future. But scientific knowledge has expanded so much in the last quarter century that we're coming close to the threshold of the Austin-Sommers era. Right now, right here in our own time, blind people see spots of light with artificial eyes, while deaf people hear tones with artificial ears. Replacement arms work like real ones. Bones are made of steel and plastic. And very soon, an atomic-driven plastic heart may be implanted in a human patient.

These spare parts for humans are not just on the drawing board. They've actually been built with biomedical materials, and are being tested by real patients today.

It all began in 1939. . . .

1

CHAPTER 1...
THE ARTIFICIAL KIDNEY

JUST BEFORE THE BEGINNING OF WORLD WAR II, DR. WIL-lem J. Kolff, a young Dutch physician, was in charge of a four-bed hospital at the University of Groningen in the Netherlands. One of his patients had headaches, vomited, and could no longer see. The twenty-two-year-old man was dying slowly and miserably from kidney disease. Because his kidneys were no longer able to remove waste materials from his blood, the young man grew weaker and weaker as his body wastes accumulated inside him. Dr. Kolff felt helpless and distressed as he stood at the bedside of the sick man.

Nearby was the patient's elderly mother, wearing her best black dress and a white lace cap. Dr. Kolff was forced to tell the sobbing woman that her only son was going to die.

The young physician realized that if there were some way to remove enough of the body wastes from the patient's blood, the man's symptoms would be relieved. If his body wastes could be removed every few days, the patient might live. But at that time there was no way to save him.

Not long afterward, Dr. Kolff began to experiment with cellophane tubing, the kind used as sausage skin. He filled the tubing with a small amount of blood and attached it to a board which he rocked back and forth in a saltwater solution for half an hour. When he tested the blood, he found that almost all of the urea (a waste product) had passed through the cellophane into the salt water.

On May 10, 1940, the German armies invaded the Netherlands. When a Nazi was appointed to head the Department of Medicine at the University of Groningen, Dr. Kolff resigned in protest and moved to Kampen, becoming head internist at a small hospital. Over the next three years he continued to work on a machine which could cleanse wastes from blood, obtaining materials in secret so that the Nazis couldn't learn of his research.

When he succeeded in building a blood-cleansing, or dialysis, machine, Dr. Kolff used it to treat fifteen patients suffering from acute kidney failure. Although their symptoms were relieved by the dialysis, the fifteen patients had been so severely ill by the time they were referred to Dr. Kolff that it was too late to save most of them. Only one of the patients lived, and Dr. Kolff was the first to admit that the man might have survived without dialysis.

Then, in September 1945, the hospital admitted a patient

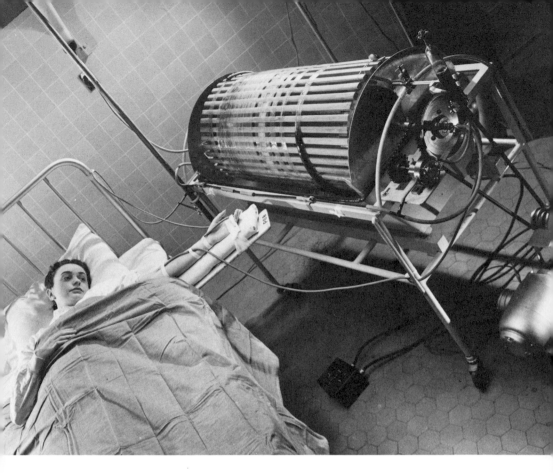

Dr. Kolff's first artificial kidney had a drum which rotated to dialyze blood.

who was in a coma because of kidney failure. The sixty-seven-year-old woman happened to be a Nazi sympathizer, completely opposed to the ideals Dr. Kolff believed in. Yet she was a patient in need of medical help, and he was a responsible physician.

When Dr. Kolff dialyzed her blood with his artificial kidney, the woman's condition improved so much that she woke up and began to speak. Because of the dialysis treatment, she eventually returned to health, becoming the first patient whose life was saved by an artificial kidney.

Dr. Kolff later came to the United States and built a more advanced model of the blood-dialyzing machine (artificial kidney). Its acceptance was slow in coming, but now, more than thirty years later, many thousands of lives have been saved because a young Dutch physician built a machine which could clean wastes from blood.

THE WAY NATURAL KIDNEYS WORK

Every normal person has two kidneys—reddish brown, bean-shaped organs located one on either side of the spine at waist level. In a grown man of average height and weight, each kidney is about 5 inches long, 2½ inches wide, 1½ inches thick, and weighs ¼ pound.

On any day, the above-mentioned healthy adult male will drink a bit less than 7 cups of liquid, and will take in 3½ cups more liquid in the food he eats. On the same day, he'll lose 3½ ounces of sweat (if the temperature is less than 70° Fahrenheit), 7 ounces of fluid in his bowel movement, 3 cups through evaporation from the lungs and skin, and 6 cups of urine. Add it up and you'll see that his intake and output are about equal. The kidneys are the organs most responsible for keeping this equilibrium.

If the weather turns really hot, our man will lose much more than 3½ ounces of perspiration. If he plays a fast game of tennis or takes part in other active exercise, he'll breathe rapidly and lose extra water vapor from his lungs. His body will respond by making him thirsty so that he'll drink more liquid, and his kidneys will respond by excreting less water in the urine. The kidneys make adjustments for wide changes inside and outside the body, and they adjust things quickly so that the body fluids stay within normal limits.

Each kidney is a complex filtration system made up of a million microscopic filters called nephrons. In each nephron, blood pressure pushes plasma (blood without red cells) through tiny, intertwined blood vessels in the part of a nephron called a glomerulus. As it passes along the tube leading from a glomerulus, the plasma moves back and forth through the tube walls, all the while being cleaned of waste materials—urea, uric acid, ammonia, creatinine, excess sodium chloride, and other substances. Materials the body still needs are returned to the blood in the capillaries surrounding the tube.

The extra water and wastes removed from the plasma become urine, and flow from the tubes into collecting ducts. Urine leaves the kidneys through the ureters, collects in the bladder, and is excreted.

To give you some idea how rapidly all this happens, the blood flow through both kidneys is 1,200 milliliters (5 cups) *each minute*. Of that amount, only $\frac{1}{10}$ is actually filtered, and even that much is not filtered completely. No single milliliter of blood has all its wastes removed in one pass through the kidney. A small amount of solute is removed from each of the many milliliters of blood flowing through each time. This may sound like a wasteful method, but it works well. 180 liters of fluid (190 quarts) are filtered each day.

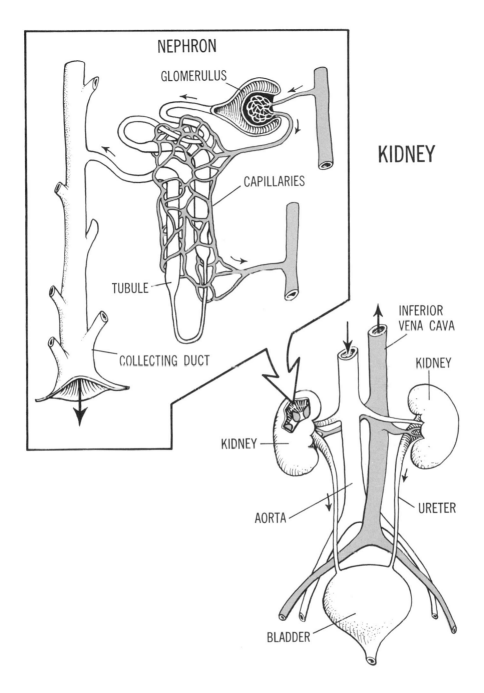

Each kidney is made up of a million microscopic filters called nephrons. Blood is cleansed of wastes as it passes through the glomerulus and tubules of a nephron.

If our man excreted 190 quarts of fluid, there'd be nothing left of him. 188 or 189 of the quarts are reabsorbed, and only 1 to 2 quarts are passed out of the body as urine. When the kidneys work properly, they make the selection—which part of the fluid is to be reabsorbed, which part is to be excreted. In this way the kidneys keep the body chemistry in fine balance.

WHEN SOMETHING GOES WRONG

A person who gets hurt in a serious accident and loses a lot of blood will go into "shock." Blood pressure will be too low to push plasma through the glomeruli in the kidneys. Since blood is the source of oxygen for all cells, the kidney cells will begin to break down due to lack of oxygen. The longer the kidneys go without oxygen, the less likely they'll be to recover when the blood pressure returns to normal. And with the kidneys not working, more and more waste material will collect inside the person's body.

The same process happens when kidneys are damaged by disease. With their own wastes building up inside them, patients will suffer from swelling of the face, hands, and legs, weakness, nausea, vomiting, high blood pressure, and eventually, death.

Before the invention of the artificial kidney, patients with acute kidney failure always died. Today, thanks to Dr. Kolff and other scientists, there are ways to cleanse or dialyze the blood to remove impurities.

HOW DIALYSIS WORKS

Why did the blood in the cellophane sausage casing become clean when Dr. Kolff rocked it in the saltwater bath?

Cellophane—which was a rather new material when Dr. Kolff began his experiments—is a thin, transparent film made from cellulose. The microscopic holes, or pores, in cellophane are so small that only small molecules can pass through them. Blood cells and proteins are too large to pass through cellophane pores, but urea and other body wastes *can* pass through them.

Concentrated molecules will always spread out, or diffuse, into a substance which does not contain many of those molecules. For instance, if you drop a lump of sugar into a cup of water, the sugar will diffuse and make the water uniformly sweet. If you hang a cellophane bag filled with salty water inside a jar of fresh water, the salt will diffuse through the pores of the cellophane until the water is equally salty inside and outside the bag. (Don't try this with a plastic bag— plastic doesn't have pores.)

In Dr. Kolff's experiment, the urea in the blood diffused through the cellophane pores into the surrounding saltwater bath, until the urea reached equilibrium (became equal) inside and out.

When a patient is on dialysis, blood is tapped from an artery in the arm or leg. The blood, pumped by the heart, flows through a tube into the artificial kidney machine, where it spreads across a membrane made of cellophane or other porous material. Depending on the type of artificial kidney used, the membrane may be tubing wrapped in a coil, sheets stacked flat, or hollow fibers. The blood-filled membrane is bathed in continuously circulating dialysis fluid. During dialysis, the fluid is changed frequently, and when enough wastes have been removed from the blood, the remaining fluid is discarded.

The patient's blood flows through the artificial kidney, and then returns to the body through a vein, making one round trip about every half hour. Dials and gauges on the machine show the temperature of fluid and blood, and indicate whether the machine is operating safely. It will turn off automatically

A patient being dialyzed by a standard artificial kidney machine. In this large model, the dialysis fluid is used, discarded and replaced in a continuous flow.

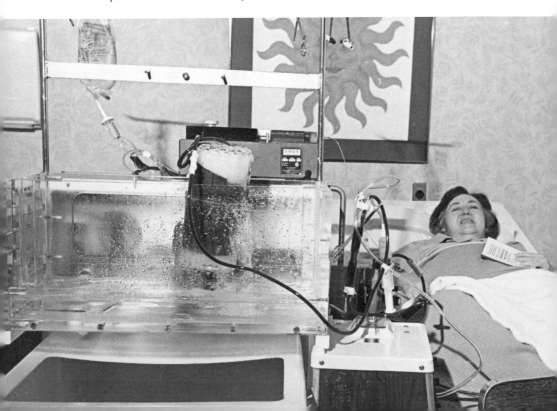

if air bubbles should get into the blood, if the blood begins to leak into the fluid, or if sterility is lost.

A patient with acute (severe) kidney disease will be admitted to a hospital where dialysis can be performed under the care of doctors and nurses until recovery. But many patients have chronic kidney disease—a condition which will never get any better and must therefore be treated again and again. Many chronic kidney patients now have artificial kidneys in their own homes. Helped by other members of their families, they're able to have their blood cleansed at home while they relax, read, or sleep. Each dialysis may last from six to ten hours, and may be performed two or three times a week.

THE PORTABLE ARTIFICIAL KIDNEY

People with healthy kidneys are having their blood cleansed constantly, every moment of their lives. If persons with diseased kidneys could have their blood cleaned continuously, they'd feel much healthier. But a patient having dialysis must be connected by tubes to a device as large as a washing machine, so he or she has to lie or sit pretty still.

Fortunately, because the body can tolerate a certain amount of buildup of wastes in the blood, kidney patients are able to go for two or three days without dialysis and still not feel too sick. How much better they'd feel, though, if they could be dialyzed daily without being attached to a large, unmovable machine; if they could move about freely and travel far from home without having to report to a dialysis center for

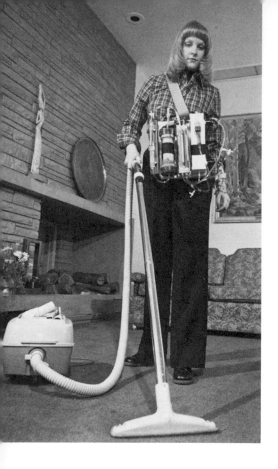

The Wearable Artificial Kidney allows patients to carry on everyday tasks while being dialyzed.

blood cleansing. Very soon now, this kind of mobility may be possible.

Dr. Willem Kolff, the scientist who invented the first workable artificial kidney, is now head of the Division of Artificial Organs at the University of Utah. Scientists at the division have built a number of artificial organs, including a portable, wearable artificial kidney called the WAK. This small dialyzer weighs eight pounds and can be carried in a case strapped across a patient's shoulder. Although they're not yet perfected enough for general use, these portable kidneys are being tried out by a number of patients.

In the WAK, a battery-powered pump draws blood through

a single needle and circulates the blood through a hollow fiber dialyzer. A separate compartment contains activated carbon which removes wastes from the dialyzing fluid. Blood returns through a Y-shaped connector back into the single needle and into the patient's body. The flow of blood is controlled by two valves which open and close rather rapidly, one in each of the two blood lines, so that blood flows through the needle in only one direction at a time.

The WAK has many advantages. It's small and lightweight, so that those using it can move freely. They can walk around, work at a desk, even travel if they want to. Because the WAK is used every day to cleanse the blood, waste products don't have a chance to build up and the patient feels much better. The WAK is less expensive to make than a standard artificial kidney, and will cost about $2,500 when produced in quantity. By contrast, home dialysis units cost anywhere from $4,000 to $10,000, while hospital dialysis costs $25,000 per year.

The WAK does have one disadvantage—as yet its activated carbon system can't remove enough urea from the blood. About every fifteen minutes the WAK must be connected to a twenty-liter tank so that more urea can be flushed out.

Patients using the WAK spend three hours a day on dialysis, and during that time the WAK is attached to the twenty-liter tank for periods totaling one and a half to two hours. Since the tank is small enough to fit under an airplane seat, people who use this system feel that it allows them much more freedom than the usual eight-hour, three-times-a-week dialysis.

A number of research projects are in progress which it is

hoped will lead to miniaturized removal systems for urea and certain other wastes. If these prove successful, a truly portable artificial kidney may not be too far away.

KIDNEY TRANSPLANTS

A healthy natural kidney will always work much better than any kind of artificial kidney. Many people who have lost the use of their own kidneys because of disease have returned to health when they received a human-kidney transplant. Since each person needs only one working kidney to stay alive and well, any healthy person can donate a kidney. Why then are artificial kidneys needed? Why can't every patient receive a kidney transplant?

First, there aren't enough donor kidneys available. Even though kidney-transplant teams in the United States have performed more than twenty-five thousand kidney transplants, there are still a great number of patients waiting for donor kidneys. The supply of donor kidneys is increasing as more people agree to donate their organs after death, but the supply can't meet the demand.

Second, kidney transplants aren't always successful. The human body will reject anything that is not a part of it. For instance, if you get a splinter in your finger, your body defense mechanisms immediately go to work to force that splinter out of your finger. Special white blood cells attack it and form a pocket of pus around it which will eventually eject the splinter. These white cells also form antibodies which attack the organisms that cause infection.

Rejection can be controlled by matching the donor organ as closely as possible to the patient receiving it—matching it by blood type, tissue pattern, and body proteins. The closer the match, the better the chance of success. Transplants between identical twins are almost always successful. Of patients who receive a kidney from a living close relative (brother or sister, parent, son or daughter) 84 percent are alive after two years.

A lower survival rate, 70 percent after two years, is found with patients who receive kidneys from cadavers, that is, from persons who have died in accidents or from other causes which did not harm their kidneys.

Certain medicines can control rejection, and persons who have received kidney transplants must take these medicines for the rest of their lives. But too much rejection-controlling medicine will weaken the body's natural defenses by suppressing the white cells that combat infection. When that happens, the patients have less resistance to disease. If they don't receive these antirejection drugs in exactly the right amount, they may die of pneumonia or from some other severe infection. And there's another problem—sometimes the transplanted kidney develops the same disease that destroyed the one which was replaced.

Many patients whose bodies reject a transplanted kidney, or who lose a transplanted kidney because it's become diseased, can stay alive with the help of an artificial kidney until another donor organ is found. About 30 percent of all kidney transplant receivers return to dialysis. It seems certain that no matter how successful kidney transplantation may become, artificial kidneys will always be needed.

CHAPTER 2...
THE ARTIFICIAL EYE

WHAT DO YOU THINK IS THE WORST THING THAT COULD HAPPEN to you? A recent Gallup poll reports that Americans are most afraid of cancer and blindness.

Fear of blindness may be due partly to superstitions that have survived since earliest times. The two-thousand-year-old Dead Sea Scrolls reveal that blind persons weren't allowed inside the temple—they were considered "unclean." In the Middle Ages, anyone who accidentally touched a blind person had to quickly say a prayer to keep from "catching" the blindness. Many people believed that blindness was a punishment for sins.

Yet blind people are ordinary people of all ages and walks of life. With proper training, they can do almost anything that sighted people can do—keep house, raise children, study, take part in sports, and work at a variety of jobs. Of course, they can't drive a cab or play pro basketball; but they swim and ski, golf and bowl, work as engineers, typists, and farmers.

In order to do all these things, blind persons must learn to move safely from place to place. But moving around without vision isn't at all easy. To try it out, cover your eyes with a blindfold and walk around a room that's familiar to you— your own bedroom or kitchen. Go to the cupboard for a glass and get yourself a drink of water from the kitchen faucet. Not so easy, but still possible. Now imagine that you're all alone on a downtown sidewalk and you can't see a thing. Strangers are hurrying past you and cars are whizzing by just beyond the curb. Without special training, you'd be completely helpless, and no doubt pretty frightened.

MOBILITY AIDS FOR THE BLIND

It's only in the past fifty years that much effort has been made to help blind people achieve mobility. In 1927 an American woman named Dorothy Harrison Eustis happened to visit a school in Germany where German shepherd dogs were being trained to guide blinded war veterans. Since Mrs. Eustis raised and trained German shepherds herself, she was very much impressed by what she saw at the school, and wrote an article about it.

After her article was published, Mrs. Eustis received a letter from twenty-year-old Morris Frank. "Thousands of blind like me hate being dependent on others," he wrote her. "Help me and I will help them. Train me and I will bring back my dog and show people here how a blind man can be absolutely on his own."

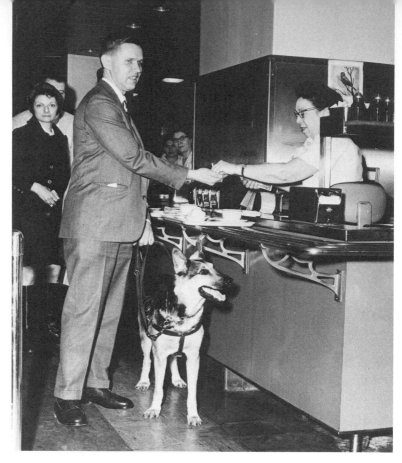

Dog guides are allowed in all public places, even where other animals aren't permitted.

Mrs. Eustis agreed. A dog was chosen for training, and Morris Frank learned to work with the dog. The two of them became such a successful team that they toured the entire country giving demonstrations of safe travel through all kinds of traffic.

In 1929 Mrs. Eustis founded The Seeing Eye, Inc., to train more dogs for the blind. Located in Morristown, New Jersey, the school has trained almost seven thousand dogs to date, and there are now eight other schools in the United States which train dog guides.

Although most of the dogs are German shepherds, other breeds can be used, such as Labrador retrievers, golden retrievers and boxers. At The Seeing Eye, about half the dogs used are bred by the organization. When the puppies are ten to twelve weeks old, they're farmed out to members of 4-H Clubs to be cared for until they're old enough for training, usually at fourteen months.

The dogs' first lessons are in obedience. They must learn to ignore all distractions, such as other dogs, cats, children, or well-meaning people who want to pat them and be friendly with them while they're working. Later they must learn to *disobey* when their owners' commands might lead to danger— for instance, if an owner signals "forward" when a car is coming.

Dog guides are allowed in all public places, even where other animals aren't permitted. They may go with their owners into restaurants, theaters, offices, or classrooms, where they lie quietly in positions that won't disturb other people. Whenever a dog is "off duty" in this way, you may pet it if the owner gives you permission. But *never* touch or talk to a dog guide when it's working or leading its owner.

Dog guides seem to be such wonderful aids for the blind that you might think every blind person would want to have one. Actually, only 1 to 2 percent of all blind people have these dogs. Some feel that taking care of a dog is too much of a chore. Others simply don't like dogs. And many feel that they can get around well enough with the most widely used mobility aid for the blind—the long cane.

Canes have been around as long as people have been

around, and blind persons have been walking with the aid of canes or staffs for centuries. But until rather recently, no one thought of trying to find out just how a blind person could use a cane most efficiently to move from place to place.

In 1930 a "white cane law" was passed giving blind persons carrying white canes the right of way at intersections. Thousands of blind persons began carrying white canes; but the canes were used mostly as a way of showing that they were blind so that others could be more careful around them. It wasn't until World War II that Dr. Richard Hoover realized that a cane would make a useful clear-path indicator to warn blind persons if something was in the way. Dr. Hoover developed a long, lightweight cane which users hold at a forward angle and move from left to right in front of them as they walk. The tip of the cane will strike anything in the way, and will warn of a curb or stairway.

ELECTRONIC MOBILITY AIDS

One thing an ordinary long cane can't do is warn of something overhead, such as a tree limb or an awning, which a blind person might unexpectedly walk into. However, a new electronic long cane, called the C-5 Laser Cane, can detect head-high objects, straight-ahead obstacles, and sudden drop-offs.

Lasers are very thin beams of light, in this case, of infrared light. Since the beams are focused so narrowly, the light's energy is highly concentrated. In the C-5 Laser Cane, one pencil-thin laser beam points upward to head height. When the beam touches a tree branch, a sign, or any overhead obstacle, it reflects back to the cane and sets off a high-pitched "beep." A center beam focuses straight ahead, up to twelve feet in front of the cane. When an obstruction is contacted by the beam, the cane sounds a middle-pitched tone. The downward-looking beam detects any drop-off lower than five inches, and causes a rasping, low-pitched sound.

It may seem to you that the C-5 Laser Cane would be simple and easy to operate, but each user has to spend between thirty and forty hours being trained to handle it correctly. And it's expensive—a Laser Cane costs $2,000. Yet users think that the time and money spent are well worth it. "You can't imagine how nice it is to be able to travel around things and people without hitting them with your cane," one woman has said.

Another brand-new mobility aid for the blind is the Sonicguide, which uses ultrasonic sound rather than a laser beam. The Sonicguide looks like a pair of ordinary eyeglasses, with frames a bit thicker than normal, and a wire running from the frame to a box which holds the power source. In the center of the eyeglass frame, just above the nose, is a transmitter which sends out a beam of ultrasonic sound waves. Ultrasonic sound has such high frequencies that it can't be heard by human ears. When this sound bounces off an object in its path, some of the sound waves are reflected back toward the person wearing the Sonicguide. Two tiny receivers, also in the nosepiece of the eyeglass frame, pick up the reflected sound. Electronic equipment in the earpieces of the glasses changes the ultrasonic sound into sound that can be heard, and feeds it through small tubes that look like hearing aids, into the ears of the wearer. These tubes transmit the electronic sounds without interfering with normal outside noises, so that the wearer can still hear conversation or traffic noises.

When the ultrasonic sound hits a hard, smooth surface, like a plate-glass window, a lot of the sound waves are reflected back. If it hits a softer, textured surface, like a person or a leafy tree, many of the sound waves are absorbed and not as many are reflected back. Because of this, differently textured objects make different noises. With training, blind persons can learn to recognize the different noises and can tell whether they're approaching a bush, a fence, a wall, or a pole. A telephone pole will sound like a repeated whistle. A bush makes a "shu, shu, shu" noise. And because sound waves reflected from the left sound louder in the left ear, and sound waves reflected from the right sound louder in the right ear, the wearer knows the position of each object ahead.

A young man who had just completed Sonicguide mobility training had to pass a "final exam." He was sent alone to a busy downtown business section and was told to locate the bus stop. This is how he handled the experience:

"As I approached the curb on the other side of the street," he says, "I lowered my head a little. I could hear the curb coming up in front of me. As I scanned [moved] my head from side to side, I could tell that there were some poles on the corner. I just headed right between those two poles. As I was walking down the sidewalk there were pedestrians coming toward me, but I could gauge my line of traffic so that I avoided them. I walked to the next corner. I could judge when I was approaching it not only by hearing the traffic, but because as I came up I could hear the feedback from the poles and the people congregating on the corner. And I noticed that the building on my side had ended because I wasn't getting feedback from the walls. Just as I approached the bus stop, a bus pulled up and the doors opened and all these people came piling off the bus. People were getting off and looking here and there where they needed to go, and talking with their friends and things like that. I didn't bump into any one of them. And I was able to hear where the metal bus pole was among all those pedestrians. It had a different sound—it had a sharp ringing sound as opposed to the 'mush mush' of the people sound."

The remarkable advancement in electronics has made possible not only mobility aids for the blind, but also some amazing new machines which help people without sight to read and to work.

The Sonicguide.

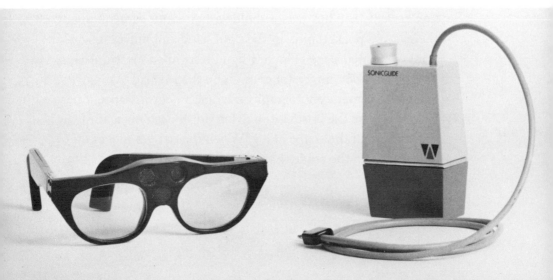

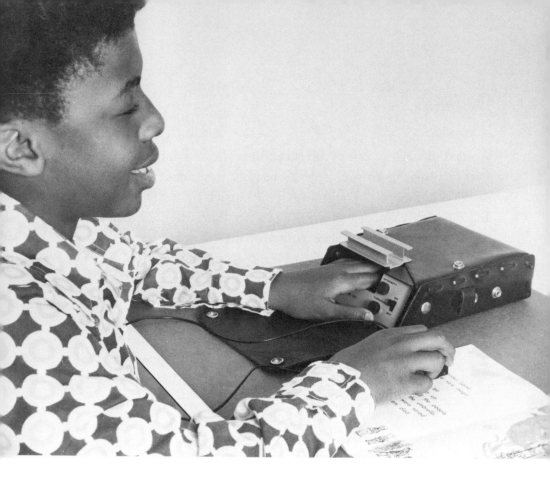

A blind student reads print with the Optacon.

The Optacon is something like a small closed-circuit television system. A blind person holds a miniature camera, about the size of a pocketknife, in the right hand and moves it slowly across a printed page. The left hand rests in an electronic box where the index finger touches a cup-shaped pad. When the hand-held camera photographs a letter, a *t* for instance, fibers which feel like the bristles of a nylon brush push up against the index finger in the shape of a *t*. When the camera moves on to an *h* and an *e*, the reader has been able to feel the word "the."

It's a slower process than reading by sight, but it allows a blind person independent access to print. Although Optacon users read at an average of forty words a minute, some have built up to speeds of eighty words a minute. The Optacon is expensive, at $2,400 per unit, but it opens the entire world of books to blind people who would otherwise be limited to bulky Braille editions, when they're available.

Another useful tool for the sightless is the talking calculator. The talking calculator has a twenty-four-word vocabulary —each key is connected to a tape recording which speaks out loud when it's pressed. After the users have learned the positions of the number and function keys on the calculator, they can feed any math problem into it. They know that they've pressed the right buttons because each number, and then the answer, is spoken aloud. The talking calculator will say "two times two equals four" or "one zero zero divided by eight

The talking calculator.

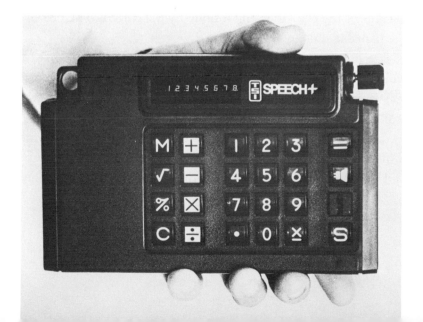

equals one two point five" in a voice that sounds like the robot from "Lost In Space."

All the above-mentioned mobility aids and work aids for the blind are substitutes for vision through the use of other senses—touch and hearing. But what if the blind could actually "see" obstacles in their paths, or see well enough to read print? Research is taking place right now on a device which would allow the blind to perceive actual images. The device is called the artificial eye, and it works by stimulating the visual cortex area of the brain. In order to understand how the artificial eye works, it will be necessary for you to understand how the natural eye works.

HOW THE NATURAL EYE WORKS

For vision to take place, light must be present. Light rays travel in straight lines to the eye, where they meet the cornea. Because the cornea is curved, as they pass through the cornea light rays are bent and angled toward each other. About 70 percent of the eye's focusing is done by the cornea. The rest of the focusing is done by the lens.

The lens is able to change shape because of the ligaments which surround and hold it. When the ligaments are taut, the lens is pulled and somewhat flattened. This happens if you're looking at something in the distance, and the lens doesn't have to do any fine focusing. However, when you want to look at something close, the ligaments relax and the lens bunches up and becomes more curved. Since the lens is then thicker, the

EYE

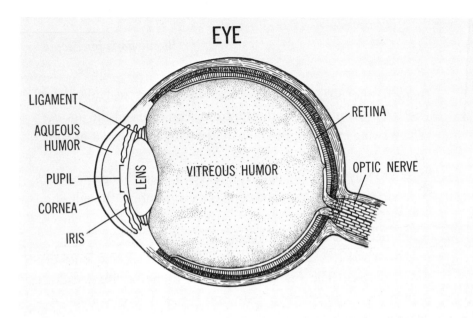

LIGAMENT

AQUEOUS HUMOR

PUPIL

CORNEA

IRIS

LENS

VITREOUS HUMOR

RETINA

OPTIC NERVE

An image is focused as it passes through the cornea and lens. At the retina, the visual function changes from mechanical to electro-chemical.

light rays are bent to a greater angle so that sharp focusing can take place.

Because both the cornea and the lens are curved, light rays passing through them are angled toward each other in the shape of a cone, and come together in a point. Past the point, the light rays fan out again into another cone going in the opposite direction. But now the light rays are upside-down and left-to-right reversed from the way they were when they entered the eye. And it's in this direction that they reach the retina.

If you are looking at a tree with a swing hanging on its left branch, the image which reaches your retina will have the tree's leaves on the bottom, the ground on top, and the upside-down swing on the right. This image will be corrected in your brain.

Up to this point, the light rays haven't been changed except to be focused. Once the image reaches your retina, though, the second part of vision begins as the visual function changes from mechanical to electrochemical.

The retina is a membrane only $\frac{1}{50}$ inch thick, made up of several layers. The first layers consist of nerve fibers called bipolar cells and ganglion cells, and the next layer is made of nerve cells called rods and cones because of the way they're shaped. When a light image reaches the retina, it passes through the bipolar cells and ganglion cells and activates the rods and cones.

Rods work in dim light and react to images in shades of gray. Cones work in brighter light and react to color. Each cone can react to only one color—either red, green, or blue. When you see orange, yellow, purple, brown, or any other color variation, it's because the cones are working together, combining and overlapping their red, green, and blue color reactions. In a similar way, you can produce any color of light by correctly combining red, green, and blue light.

The rods and cones contain chemicals which are changed by light. These chemicals break down when light touches them, exciting a signal which jumps to the bipolar cells. The bipolar cells react and cause a signal which crosses to the ganglion cells, which also react. The axons, or long, thin "tails" of the ganglion cells, come together to form a bundle which is known as the optic nerve.

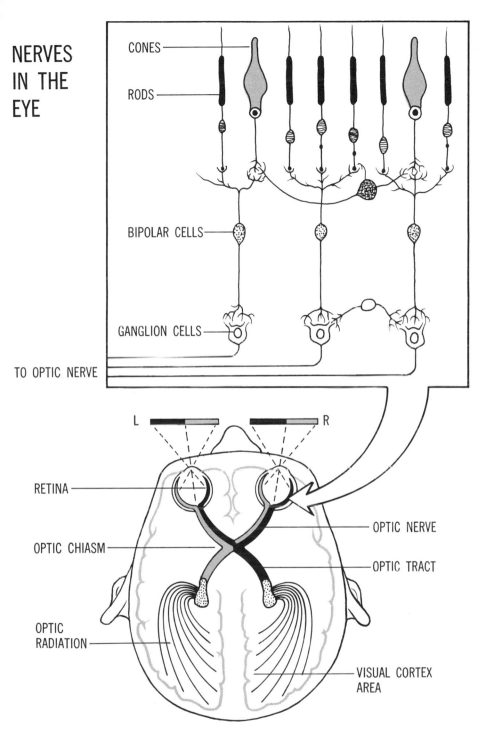

NERVES IN THE EYE

CONES

RODS

BIPOLAR CELLS

GANGLION CELLS

TO OPTIC NERVE

L   R

RETINA

OPTIC CHIASM

OPTIC RADIATION

OPTIC NERVE

OPTIC TRACT

VISUAL CORTEX AREA

From the nerve cells of the retina, visual signals travel through the optic nerves, optic tracts, and optic radiations to the visual cortex area of the brain.

The optic nerves leave the back of the eye and travel into the brain. But they don't go straight back; they turn inward toward the center of the brain. Where they meet, the bundles divide in two and cross each other at a point known as the optic chiasm. Behind the optic chiasm, the nerve fibers are called optic tracts. The optic tracts regroup into new nerve bundles in the thalamus of the brain. From this point on, the nerve fibers are not so close together—they're more spread out. The visual cortex is located at the lower part of the back of the brain, in small areas just to the left and the right of the division between the two halves of the brain.

When a visual impulse travels through the optic nerves, the optic tracts, and the more loosely packed optic radiations, it fires a series of signals to the cells in the visual cortex of the brain. As the cells of the visual cortex react, you see an image. This whole process takes place in not much more than $\frac{1}{100}$ second.

The visual cortex area of the brain can be damaged by a stroke, a tumor, or an injury. If your visual cortex is damaged, you won't be able to see, even though your eyes and visual pathways are working.

HOW ARTIFICIAL VISION WORKS

In 1968, two English scientists, Giles Brindley and Walpole Lewin, placed an array of eighty-one electrodes inside the skull and against the right visual cortex of a fifty-two-year-old blind woman. (An array means a series of rows. An electrode is a wire through which an electric current passes.) When the woman's visual cortex was stimulated by weak electrical current, she saw small dots of light, similar to the spots of light you see if you rub your eyes too hard, or if you receive a blow on the head and "see stars." These spots of light which resulted from the experiment were named phosphenes.

Scientists at the University of Utah's Division of Artificial Organs wondered whether Dr. Brindley's experiment might lead to a useful device for the blind. They decided to develop a device that would use phosphenes to produce a substitute for real sight, one that might allow a blind person to recognize objects and to move about safely. In 1969 a research team was organized by Dr. William Dobelle to begin work on the project.

The team hopes to eventually create an artificial eye using a miniature TV camera and a tiny computer. The camera would be fitted into a glass eye, which would be placed into a blind patient's eye socket and attached to eye muscles, allowing it to move the way a normal eye moves. The camera in the glass eye would send electrical signals through wires to a tiny computer contained in an eyeglass frame. These signals would then be translated, by the computer, into information sent through wires running to electrodes on the visual cortex of the brain.

When the team began its work, it faced a difficult task. Designing the tiny camera and computer would be hard enough; but many questions had to be answered before the actual experiments could begin. For example, how does the visual cortex behave after a person has been blind for many

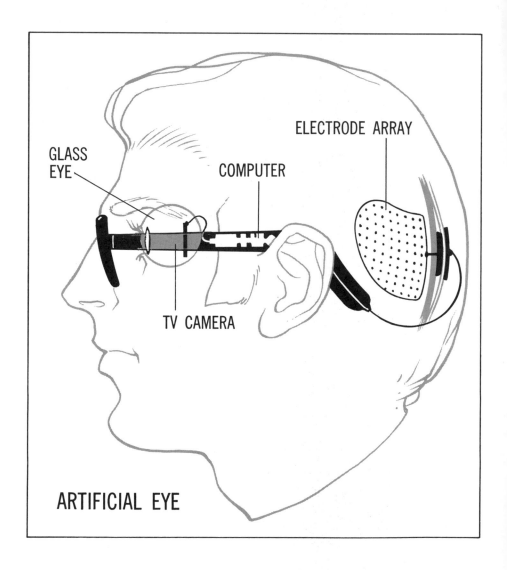

When artificial vision becomes perfected, a small TV camera will be connected through a subminiature computer to electrodes on the brain's visual cortex.

years—does it remain the same as in sighted persons, or do the nerve cells rearrange themselves because they're not being used? If Dr. Brindley's findings were typical for all blind people, could phosphenes be organized into patterns, even simple patterns such as a triangle or a square? What would happen to the brain after many years of stimulation with weak currents of electricity? And, because the chemicals in the human body can damage many plastics, metals, and other materials over a period of time, what substances should be used to make the electrodes which would be placed inside a patient's skull?

Some members of the team began looking for materials that would not damage the brain or be damaged by the body. Others, under the direction of Dr. Mike Mladejovsky, began to design a computer and the electrodes which would be needed later for experiments with blind volunteers.

Meanwhile, Dr. Dobelle and other members of the team set out to discover how the visual cortex reacts in sighted persons. Surgeons throughout the United States and Canada were asked to notify the team whenever a patient had a brain tumor in the region of the visual cortex. If the patient agreed to take part in an experiment, the team and its equipment would be flown to the city where the operation was to take place.

Before the surgeon removed the tumor, the researchers placed electrodes against the exposed visual cortex of the patient, and stimulated the brain cells with short pulses of electricity. The patient would see spots of light, and would tell the researchers where the spots appeared to be—straight ahead, to the left, to the right, and so on. (Because the brain does not experience pain, the patients were able to be awake during the experiments.)

After thirty-seven of these experiments, the research team learned some important facts about how phosphenes behave in sighted people (all thirty-seven patients had normal vision). If electricity was passed through only one electrode, the patient usually saw only one phosphene. This phosphene would become brighter or dimmer depending on the strength of the current passing through the electrode. When a patient moved his or her eyes, the phosphenes moved, too, but they always remained in the same position relative to one another.

By this time, the computer and other pieces of equipment were ready for brief experiments on blind patients. For several years, two volunteers named Dave and Doug had attended workshops at the University of Utah, learning about the research program. Dave was a forty-three-year-old piano tuner who had been blind for twenty-eight years. Doug, who had lost his sight in a land-mine explosion in Vietnam, was twenty-nine.

In early autumn of 1973, Dave, Doug, and the team flew with the new equipment to Ontario, Canada. Operations on both men were performed at the same time by Dr. John Girvin, a brain surgeon at the University of Western Ontario, who was assisted by neurosurgeon Dr. Ted Roberts from the University of Utah.

First Dr. Girvin made a small opening in the skull and slipped a ribbon-shaped piece of Teflon through the opening so that it rested against the visual cortex. Embedded in this Teflon ribbon were sixty-four electrodes and connecting wires. He then closed the opening so that only the Teflon ribbon protruded through the skin. The wires leading from the electrodes were connected to a large computer programmed to select phosphenes which would form patterns.

During three days of experiments, the electrodes were activated, and Dave and Doug described what they saw. When more than one electrode was activated, Doug could see phosphene patterns in the shapes of squares, triangles, or simple letters. Because Dave's array had slipped a bit, he couldn't see patterns, but he could still see spots of light. This was an important finding, because Dave had been without sight for twenty-eight years. It indicated that even people blind for a long time might be able to use the artificial eye device.

After three days, Dr. Girvin removed the electrodes from Dave and Doug, and shortly afterward the men were able to leave the hospital. At this point, the research team felt the need to work with a long-term implant, so that increased amounts of information could be gathered.

Craig, a man blinded by gunshot ten years earlier, volunteered to take part in the experiment. Like Dave and Doug, he had trained in the program for a long time. Again, Dr. Girvin and Dr. Roberts performed the surgery, but Craig's operation was somewhat different from Dave's or Doug's. The Teflon ribbon containing the connecting wires does not protrude through Craig's skin. Instead, the ribbon ends in a small graphite button about the size of a dime, which is attached to his skull under the skin above his right ear. Only a small portion of this button, or connector, shows through his skin, and it is normally covered by his hair. Whenever Craig participates in tests, the wires from the computer are connected, through the button, to wires leading to his electrodes.

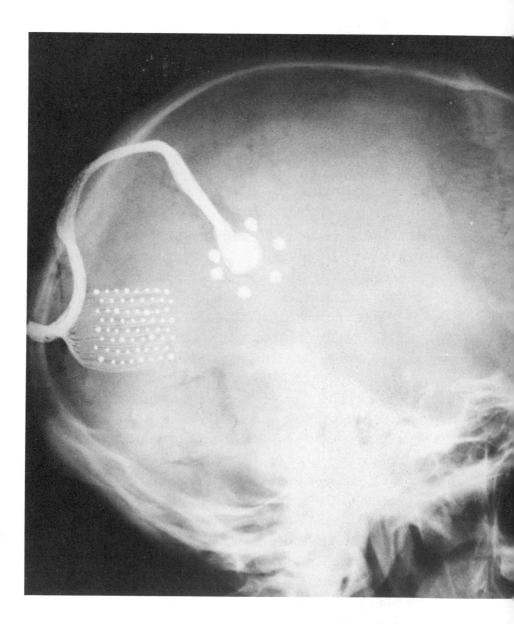

Skull X ray showing the 64 electrodes in Craig's implant.

Even though the electrodes in Craig's array are lined up in neat rows, the phosphenes that he sees do *not* appear in neat rows. If three electrodes in a straight line are activated at the same time, Craig might describe them like this: "The second one is above the first one. The third one is below the first one and to the left." If the positions of all sixty phosphenes (four connecting wires have broken, so only sixty of the original sixty-four electrodes are working) were marked on a piece of paper, they would look like a spray of buckshot.

Because each person's brain is slightly different from everyone else's, and because electrode arrays cannot be placed in precisely the same spot on the visual cortex of each blind volunteer, electrode arrays in future volunteers will produce phosphenes in different positions from Craig's. For this reason, each phosphene will have to be mapped with every patient who receives a visual cortex implant. Fortunately, the phosphenes don't change positions once they're mapped. Each time electrode number 1, 2, 3, or whatever is activated in Craig's array, the phosphene it creates appears in the same place to him.

Having learned the positions of Craig's sixty phosphenes, the team is able to send patterns to him. But because sixty electrodes aren't enough to clearly outline all twenty-six letters of the alphabet, the team uses Braille letters, which can be formed with only six points of light. Before the implant, Craig knew how to use Braille by touch, but he wasn't a very fast Braille reader. Now, when he sees Braille letters formed by phosphenes, he's able to read them much faster than he can by touch.

After two years, Craig had not suffered any ill effects from the experiments or from his electrodes. Dr. Dobelle and his team are planning to implant electrodes in other blind volunteers. Research on artificial vision is also being carried on at Maudsley Hospital in South London, under the direction of Dr. Brindley.

In the future, perhaps as many as 256 electrodes will be implanted on both the left and right visual cortex areas. As more and more phosphenes are produced, images transmitted from the camera that the researchers hope to design should look like the pictures sent to earth by the first astronauts on the moon. The images will be made up of many dots with shadings in several tones of gray. Artificial eye users won't be able to see fine detail the way a sighted person can, but they should be able to see shapes, to recognize faces, and to read at a useful speed.

It will take many years to learn exactly how the visual cortex behaves in blind people, and to perfect a wearable artificial eye. If and when the artificial eye is developed and becomes available to blind persons, they'll be able to function much more comfortably in a world of sighted people.

CHAPTER 3...
THE ARTIFICIAL EAR

Would you rather be blind or deaf?

Of course you'd rather be neither, but if you had to choose between the two handicaps, you'd probably choose deafness. After all, not being able to see is a lot worse than not being able to hear, isn't it? A blind person can never gaze on the face of a loved one, or read a book the way you can, or watch television, or marvel at a sunset. Deaf persons can do all those things. They just can't hear.

It may surprise you to learn that many people consider deafness a far greater handicap than blindness. Helen Keller, the remarkable woman who could neither see nor hear, wrote, "The problems of deafness are deeper and more complex, if not more important, than those of blindness. Deafness is a much worse misfortune. . . .

"Ours is not the silence that soothes the weary senses," Miss Keller added. "It is an inhuman silence which severs and estranges. It is a silence which isolates, cruelly and completely. Hearing is the deepest, most humanizing, philosophical sense man possesses."

Without hearing, there can be no communication. Imagine that you suddenly found yourself in a market place in Pakistan. All around you people were talking and shouting, caught up in buying and selling and *communicating*. All of it would be meaningless to you, because you wouldn't understand the language. Yet your isolation wouldn't be total, because you would hear voices, the rumble of buses, the clop of horses' hooves, the policeman's whistle. If someone shouted for you to get out of the way of a moving cart, you could hear the warning tone in the voice even though you didn't understand the words.

To get an idea of life in a silent world, turn on your television set without any sound. Watch the actors talking with one another, moving from place to place, touching, laughing, and crying. You won't know *why* they are doing any of these things, because you can't hear the words which explain their actions.

BORN DEAF

From the moment children with normal hearing are born, they begin to hear sounds which explain the world around them—the mother's voice, her footsteps, their own cries when they're hungry or uncomfortable. In the first few months of life they learn to identify these sounds, and by the end of the first year they are trying to say words—"Mama, Dada, bye-bye." By the age of two they can make themselves understood —"Want a cookie. Finger hurt. Go outside."

A child born deaf hears none of these sounds. The deaf child doesn't know that there are such things as words. The mother's warning shout that the stairs are dangerous goes unheeded because it's unheard. How can a deaf child explain that a favorite toy is lost when he or she doesn't know the word for toy, having never heard it? The sounds deaf children make are meaningless, if they bother to make any sounds at all.

They not only can't talk, they can hardly think! Words are the building blocks of reasoning. Without words, a person may communicate with gestures, but that kind of communication will remain on a very primitive level.

If a child's deafness is discovered in infancy, the parents can begin training him or her to communicate. The earlier this training begins, the better the child will be able to adjust to the normal world. The first two years of life are extremely important to the development of the language centers of the brain. If a child can't hear, the nerve pathways which link sound to language and learning will fail to develop properly. If training is delayed until the age of three or four, the child will never be able to catch up completely.

The first step is to fit the deaf baby with a hearing aid. Hearing aids do nothing except amplify sound, making it louder. Almost every deaf person has some amount of hearing, although it may be very small—what to you is a very loud shout would be barely perceptible to a deaf person. With a hearing aid to amplify sound to the greatest degree possible, a child can begin to respond with that "residual" hearing to the few things he or she is able to hear—a door slamming, a very loud bell, a warning cry.

Most tiny children react with joy and wonder when they hear a recognizable sound for the very first time. In her autobiography, *Bubbles*, Beverly Sills writes about her daughter Muffy. "One day she moved close to a hot stove and I grabbed her in time, screaming HOT! HOT! HOT! She spent the rest of the day wandering around the house saying hot, hot to everyone, her face lit up with a smile. It was the first word she had ever spoken." Prior to this incident, Muffy's parents hadn't realized that she had a profound hearing loss.

For deaf children to respond to the best of their ability to the world around them, their parents must be willing to work very hard. A single word may have to be repeated thousands of times before the deaf child understands what it means. When they are three or four years old, if they're lucky enough to live where there's a school for the deaf they can begin to attend special classes taught by highly trained teachers.

All schools for the deaf are not the same. Some concentrate on teaching a child to speak as normally as possible; to hear as much as possible with a hearing aid; and to read lips, which is called speechreading. This program is called oral communication.

Other schools teach total communication which includes

the oral skills mentioned above, but adds sign language. Total-communication teachers believe that oral training by itself is too hard and frustrating for a child to manage. They think that a deaf child should be able to communicate in the easiest possible way—by signs and gestures—so that he or she won't feel so isolated while struggling to learn the skills of oral communication. They say that being able to both sign and speak is an advantage, like being able to talk in two languages.

Oral-communication supporters believe that if children are allowed to communicate with signs and gestures, they won't be motivated to talk and speechread. They say that because deaf people must learn to live in a world of people who speak and hear, a child who learns to speak and read lips from the very beginning will adjust better to the hearing world.

All schools for the deaf have electronic devices to help the children hear the teacher and the classroom sounds. With powerful hearing aids, deaf children may be able to hear some sounds, but they hear them very differently than you would. With no effort, you learned to recognize the school bell. Deaf children must be taught to identify the slight noise they hear when the bell is rung.

Even a deaf person who has enough hearing ability to hear a voice isn't able to distinguish words the way you do. If someone says, "Hang up your coat," the deaf person may hear only the vowels—ă-oo-oh—which are strong sounds that come through loudest. The *h* may not be heard because it is made with the breath rather than the voice. *P, c,* and *t* are breath sounds like *h.*

If a deaf adult reads lips well, he or she may recognize some of the words in a sentence, and be able to fill in the rest mentally. Since deaf children haven't had much experience with language, it takes years of practice to combine the sounds they hear with the shape of words on a speaker's lips so that they can understand speech. And even when they recognize the words, deaf children miss the differences in tones which carry so much meaning.

Although many deaf persons learn to speak very well, their speech sounds different from yours because they can't hear themselves well enough to control the way they sound. If you should become deaf right now, even though you've been talking normally for years your speech would eventually change, because if you can't hear yourself, you tend to relax your vocal mechanism. You might speak too softly, simply because you couldn't hear background noise and wouldn't know that you must raise your voice to be heard in a noisy room. Or you might shout too loudly, because you're unable to gauge the volume of your own voice. And your speech would become monotonous and flat.

Your brain is constantly receiving auditory information, even when you aren't aware of it. You may be all alone in a house that seems quiet. Although you don't perceive any sounds because you're not paying attention, your ears pick up the hum of the refrigerator, the drip of a faucet, the ticking of the clock, the thump of your dog's tail. Each of these noises carries information to your mind, information which you consciously ignore but unconsciously notice. A deaf person misses all this auditory input.

HEARING AIDS

There are not as many devices to help the deaf as there are to help the blind. The best-known is the hearing aid, which has been available for decades. With the advance of electronics, hearing aids are becoming smaller but more powerful.

An in-the-ear hearing aid looks like a button, and has a receiver which works like the speaker of a radio. It's useful for mild hearing loss.

A behind-the-ear aid has a microphone, an amplifier, and a receiver in a single unit which is connected to an ear mold by a short plastic tube. The ear mold is a piece of plastic shaped to the contour of the ear to form a seal, so that no sound can leak out. One type of hearing aid is built into eyeglass frames, with a plastic tube leading from the frame into the ear.

Another type of hearing aid is called a body aid because it has a larger microphone, amplifier, and power supply packed in a case which can be worn in a pocket or strapped to the chest. A cord runs from the case to the ear mold. People who have severe hearing loss wear the body aid because it's more powerful, and many deaf persons wear two aids, one in each ear.

Although there are a number of devices to aid the hard-of-hearing, they don't seem to be as technically complex as the mobility aids for the blind. A few of them are:

The Waker-Upper, for persons who can't hear an alarm clock ring. Tucked under the bed pillow, this small device is wired to an alarm clock, and vibrates to wake a sleeper at the proper time.

The Signalman is a unit for those who can't hear a telephone bell. Any lamp, when plugged into the unit, will flash on and off each time the phone rings. For someone who is both blind and deaf, a small electric fan will signal the phone's ringing by gently blowing air toward the person.

The Silent Pager provides a way for parents of deaf children to contact them. Similar to a hospital beeper, it emits a series of silent, pulsed vibrations, alerting the child to return home. The parent can activate the pager by dialing a special telephone number.

Voice-Lite is a pyramid-shaped box with a large light on top. It's used to help deaf and speech-impaired persons learn to talk clearly. If the patient speaks with a soft, short sound, the dome of the Voice-Lite will light briefly and dimly. A long, loud sound will produce a bright light which remains on until the sound stops.

Pho-Vi (phonic-visual) Cards feature photographs of thirty-four lip and tongue positions representing the speech sounds of the English language. Like flash cards for reading and math, the Pho-Vi cards can be held up to show children the correct way to shape their lips to make a particular sound. They're also useful for teaching speechreading.

HEARING DOGS

In 1973 Mrs. Elva Janke lost her dog. The loss was very serious for Mrs. Janke because she is deaf, and she had trained her dog to respond to the sounds she couldn't hear. Mrs. Janke felt that she was too old to begin training another dog, so she asked the Minnesota Society to Prevent Cruelty (SPC) for help.

Ruth Deschene, a director for the Minnesota SPC, became interested in the idea of dogs hearing for deaf people. She brought together rehabilitation experts, obedience trainers, and members of deaf persons' groups to begin an animal-training program.

They started with six dogs, four of them homeless mongrels from animal shelters. "The dogs don't have to be purebred animals," Mrs. Deschene explained, "just young, alert, housebroken, and ready for obedience training."

After they learn obedience, the dogs are taught to respond to hand signals. Then they learn to recognize the sounds made by alarm clocks and smoke alarms, car horns, doorbells, ringing telephones, and crying children. When a trained dog hears these noises, it nudges its master, runs to the source of the sound, and returns to its master.

It takes less time to teach a hearing dog than a guide dog for the blind, and any size or breed can be used. "The training is totally different from obedience training," one dog expert has said. "It involves a happy type of training—all praise— keeping the dog happy all the time and making a game of the tasks." And a rehabilitation counselor states, "Although the program is experimental, the most exciting thing about it is that it does work and offers unlimited potential to deaf employees both at home and at work. In the future, hearing dogs may be as common and accepted in business situations as are Seeing Eye dogs."

Hearing dogs are now being trained in Denver, Colorado, at the headquarters of the American Humane Association.

HOW THE NATURAL EAR WORKS

In order to understand how artificial hearing works, you must know how the normal ear functions; and before you can understand normal hearing, you must learn something about sound.

All sound is caused by vibration. To watch it happen, cut an elastic band and tie one end around a doorknob. Stretch the elastic, and pluck it to make it vibrate and hum.

As the elastic moves up, it forces air molecules next to it to move up also. These molecules push the molecules next to them, and so on, creating a region of high pressure in which the molecules are close together. When the elastic band has gone as far as its momentum takes it, it bounces back, pulling apart the molecules behind it, causing an area of low pressure. Since the elastic band is moving back and forth very rapidly, it's causing a number of areas of high and low pressure on both sides of it, with disturbances traveling from one molecule to another in a pattern of high-pressure and low-pressure waves. It is through these waves that sound travels.

The vibrations of the elastic band have created the sound you hear. The sound of a drumbeat is caused by the vibration of the drum head, and the sound of your voice comes from the vibration of your vocal cords. If you put your hand over your throat while you're speaking, you can feel the vibrations.

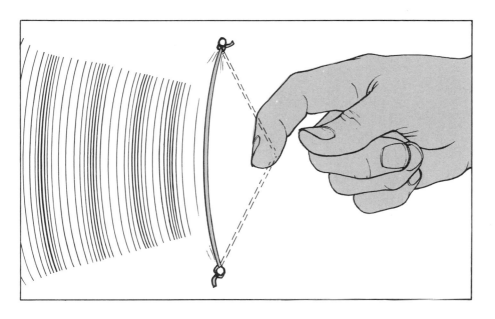

A vibrating elastic band creates a pattern of high-pressure and low-pressure waves through which sound travels.

A single vibration—one movement up and one down—is called a cycle. The number of cycles that something vibrates in a second is called its frequency. If the elastic band vibrates seventy times in a second, it has a frequency of seventy cycles per second. The highness or lowness of a tone is called its pitch, and the higher the frequency, the higher the pitch. In other words, if something vibrates slowly, it has a low sound (frequency, pitch), and if it vibrates rapidly, it has a high sound (frequency, pitch).

For example, if you have an electric blender at home, turn it on at its lowest speed, then push the buttons to make it go faster and faster. You'll notice that the sound it makes rises higher and higher, from a rumble to a whine. When it's at the highest speed, turn it off, and you'll hear the pitch descend as the motor slows down and stops. On a much larger scale, listen to the sound of a jet plane in an airport as its engines warm up from a roar to a scream. The faster the vibrations, the higher the frequency. The human ear can hear frequencies from thirty cycles per second to twenty thousand cycles per second.

Most of the sound waves you hear have traveled to your

All sound is made by vibration. Slow vibrations cause low-pitched sounds and rapid vibrations cause high-pitched sounds.

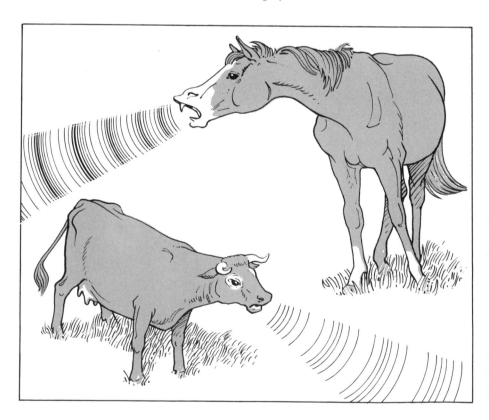

ears through the air around you. When a sound wave reaches the outer ear, it is channeled through the auditory canal to the eardrum. The pressure of the sound wave makes the eardrum vibrate—slowly for a low-frequency sound, faster for a high-frequency sound.

When the eardrum vibrates, it pushes against the hammer, which is attached to the inner side of the eardrum. The hammer is tied by tiny ligaments to the anvil, which is attached to the stirrup, so that all three bones move together. The end of the stirrup pushes on the oval window. Because the oval window is much smaller than the eardrum, and because the three bones pushing together act as levers, the pressure reaching the oval window is twenty-two times greater than it was on the eardrum. This extra pressure is needed because the inner ear is filled with fluid, and it's harder to move fluid than air.

The cochlea of the inner ear is a spiral, wound two and a half times around a tiny pillar of bone. The entire cochlea is no bigger than a pea, and the part of the skull which protects it is the thickest, hardest bone in the human body. If the cochlea were unwound, it would be 1½ inches long. It's divided by the basilar membrane, which is made up of from twenty to twenty-five thousand strands of fiber. Each basilar fiber can vibrate because it's attached at one end and free at the other end.

When the stirrup pushes on the oval window, a fluid pressure wave runs along the basilar membrane like a ripple on the surface of a pond. If a high-frequency sound wave has produced the fluid pressure wave, the fluid wave will travel just a short distance along the basilar membrane. There it will

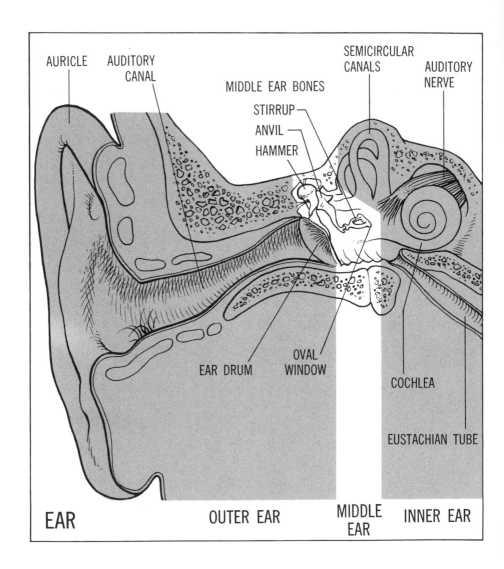

AURICLE   AUDITORY CANAL

SEMICIRCULAR CANALS   AUDITORY NERVE

MIDDLE EAR BONES

STIRRUP

ANVIL

HAMMER

EAR DRUM

OVAL WINDOW

COCHLEA

EUSTACHIAN TUBE

EAR   OUTER EAR   MIDDLE EAR   INNER EAR

Sound is channeled through the auditory canal to the eardrum which moves the bones of the middle ear. The most important part of the hearing mechanism is in the inner ear.

INTERIOR OF COCHLEA

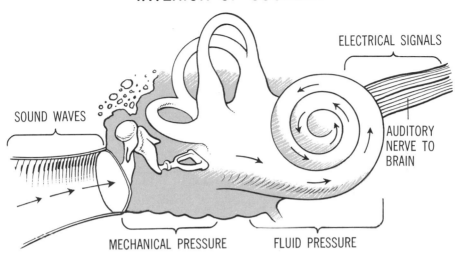

ELECTRICAL SIGNALS

SOUND WAVES

AUDITORY NERVE TO BRAIN

MECHANICAL PRESSURE

FLUID PRESSURE

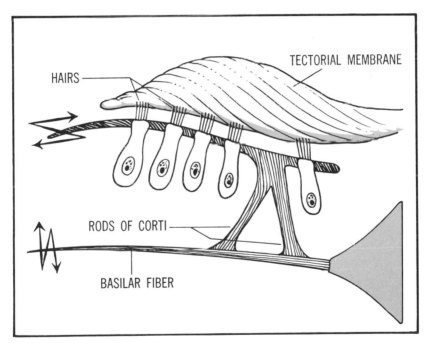

TECTORIAL MEMBRANE

HAIRS

RODS OF CORTI

BASILAR FIBER

As sound waves move through the parts of the ear, they change from mechanical energy to fluid pressure waves to electrical impulses. The bending motion of hair cells fires the nerve fibers.

rise to a peak and die out. A fluid wave from a medium-frequency sound wave will peak about halfway along the basilar membrane, and one from a low-frequency sound will travel to the end. The final force of the wave spends itself against the round window.

Resting on the basilar membrane is the organ of Corti. It contains twenty-three thousand five hundred hair cells topped by fine soft hairs. The tips of these hairs are held fast in another membrane called the tectorial membrane.

When a fluid pressure wave vibrates the basilar fibers, they in turn move the hair cells. The tiny hairs topping the hair cells can't move freely, because they're caught in the tectorial membrane. But they do bend back and forth, and this motion causes electrical signals which fire the nerve fibers at the base of the hair cells. At this point, sound waves have changed from mechanical energy to fluid pressure waves to electrical impulses.

If a sound is very loud, the nerve cells fire at a faster rate, more nerve cells fire, and certain hair cells are stimulated which only react to loud noise. Different pitches cause reactions in different bunches of hair cells, corresponding to the part of the basilar membrane where the fluid pressure wave peaked.

The nerve fibers are grouped according to the frequencies of the signals they carry. These nerve fibers lead away from the organ of Corti to form the auditory nerve. They carry only electrical signals, not the sounds themselves. It will be up to the brain to interpret the electrical signals as sounds.

Just as no one knows exactly how the brain interprets visual signals as images, no one yet knows how the brain interprets the electrical signals from the auditory nerves as sound. The auditory nerves travel an extremely complicated path from both inner ears through the brain, dividing, regrouping, and passing through several relay stations on the way. They arrive at the hearing center of the brain (auditory cortex areas), which are just above your ears.

WHEN SOMETHING GOES WRONG

There are two types of hearing loss: conductive deafness, in which something is wrong with the outer or middle ear; and nerve deafness, in which something is wrong with the inner ear or the auditory nerve. Conductive deafness can sometimes be corrected by medical treatment or surgery: nerve deafness cannot. Both can be helped to some extent by hearing aids.

The ideal hearing device would bypass the faulty parts of the ear, and work directly on the inner ear. Or, if the inner ear was damaged, it would work on the auditory cortex areas. Devices of this kind are being researched right now.

COCHLEAR IMPLANTS

In the late 1950s, Dr. William F. House was practicing medicine in California, specializing in problems of the deaf. A patient brought to his attention a newspaper account of work that researchers had done earlier on a cochlear implant. The article was optimistic about possible benefits that might be achieved through electrical stimulation of the inner ear. At that time there was still a lot of doubt about the safety of inserting anything into the inner ear, but the prospect of cochlear implants was an exciting one.

Dr. House began observing the electrical activity of the acoustic nerve when an electrode was placed on the nerve during surgery. He conducted animal studies, and over the next decade he developed more sophisticated systems with the help of his engineer, Jack Urban. Working at the Ear Research Institute in Los Angeles, Dr. House then proceeded to insert cochlear implants in long-term patients. About twenty patients now have the cochlear implants, which are put into place through the round window of the cochlea.

The first long-term subject was Charles Graser, a California teacher who had previously driven a tank truck on weekends. One day in 1959 when he was refueling a truck, it burst into flames which burned him badly. While he was hospitalized for treatment of the burns, Mr. Graser took large doeses of antibiotics to combat infection and high fevers. Unfortunately, the antibiotics destroyed the hair cells in the cochleas of his inner ears.

For many years Mr. Graser was completely deaf. He wore hearing aids, but they gave extremely limited help because his hair cells didn't function. Then, in 1970, Dr. House implanted five platinum electrodes into Mr. Graser's cochlea. The wires from the electrodes ran to a plug behind Mr. Graser's ear, and the plug picked up signals from a transmitter at the end of his eyeglass temple piece. A cord connected the transmitter to a

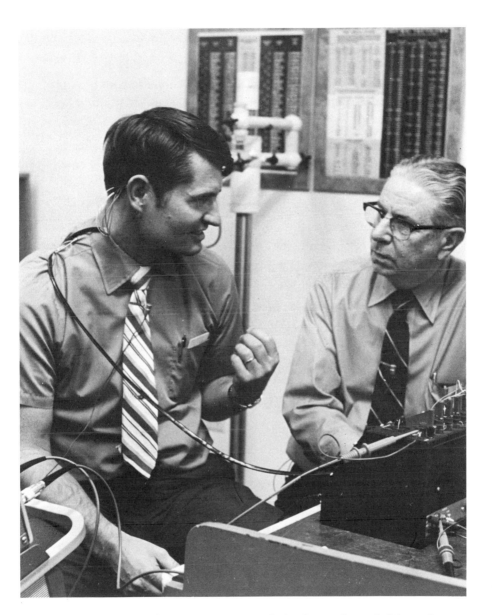

Charles Graser (left) reacts to sounds he hears through his cochlear implant during a testing session.

battery-operated receiver worn on his chest. Sounds picked up
by the receiver were converted to electric signals sent through
the wires to the points of the electrodes implanted in his
cochlea.

Mr. Graser's implant is still functioning. It enables him to
hear environmental sounds, and it helps him to recognize
speech patterns. He can't hear enough to discriminate speech
in a conversation, but he can understand simple sentences just
from the rhythm, or tempo, of the words. Being able to hear
the rhythm of speech helps him to read lips more easily.

At the University of Utah, researchers are using a computer
to transform incoming sound into signals that can be used in
artificial hearing. Working with two experimental subjects,
they've placed five or six electrodes inside the cochlea from its
base (beginning) to its tip. In laboratory experiments, when
the electrode nearest the base of the cochlea is stimulated
electrically, the patient hears a higher-pitched sound than
when an electrode near the tip of the cochlea is stimulated.
This is what you would expect, if you remember that in normal hearing higher-frequency fluid pressure waves peak nearer
the base of the cochlea.

The researchers have also tested single electrodes at different frequencies. When an electrode is stimulated at 400 cycles
per second, the patient hears a higher-pitched sound than at
100 cycles per second, confirming Dr. House's early work.
Researchers at the University of Utah are now trying to make
more complex sounds by stimulating more than one electrode
at a time, and by using several frequencies at a time. They
hope that, in the future, cochlear implants with larger num-

COCHLEAR IMPLANT

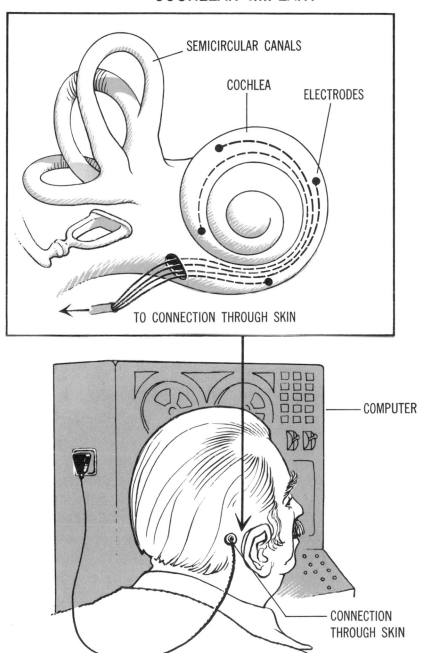

A computerized, multi-channel cochlear implant may allow deaf patients to discriminate pitch and understand speech. In future use, the computer will be miniaturized.

bers of electrodes will allow deaf patients to understand speech.

To help scientists at the Ear Research Institute, a number of the patients have kept written accounts of their hearing experiences. In Charles Graser's journal, he says, "I was deaf for twelve years, but now I hear. Using this new device has reopened the world to me. I can call home from my work as the Colton High School librarian and ask my wife what she is planning for dinner or what she bought on her shopping trip. The conversation is quite restricted, but it really works. I also get tremendous enjoyment hearing the bells at school, traffic noises on the highway, a mockingbird calling, the cat meowing, bacon frying, and on and on. Now when I am camping and hear a chipmunk stealing peanuts out of the sack beside me, I know that I am no longer deaf."

THE ARTIFICIAL EAR

The artificial ear will work on the same principle as the artificial eye. Just as the artificial eye stimulates the visual cortex area of the brain, the artificial ear will stimulate the auditory cortex area. You learned in the previous chapter that when small pulses of electricity are sent to the visual cortex area of the brain, a patient sees spots of light called phosphenes. In the same way, when small pulses of electricity are sent to the auditory cortex area of the brain, a patient hears sounds. These sounds are called audcncs.

Research on the artificial ear has not gone very far because it's harder to find patients who are having surgery on that area of the brain. Also, the hearing centers are not located just on the surface of the brain, but extend farther under the surface. Stimulation of the deeper areas could create risks for the patient.

To date, eight patients who were undergoing surgery for other reasons have volunteered for auditory cortical stimulation. All of them had normal hearing, and all of them had been taught, before the operations, to notice differences in loudness and pitch. They were awake, under local anesthetic, when the experiments were performed by Drs. Dobelle and Mladejovsky and others of the team which had also developed the artificial eye.

A single, hand-held electrode was placed against the exposed auditory cortex of the patients. When an electric current was passed into the brain, the patients said they heard sound. Then the electrode would be moved to another spot in the auditory cortex, and activated again. Most times, in each location, the patients reported hearing sounds which they described as a buzz, a hum, knocking, or "crickets." If the electric current was increased, the sounds grew louder. For reasons the scientists don't yet understand, it takes twice as much current to produce audenes as it does to produce phosphenes.

With all eight patients, the electrodes were held in place only during the experiments. There were no implants. Researchers hope that in the future, a ribbon-cable array of sixty-four electrodes may be left in place for longer periods, so that audenes can be mapped the way that phosphenes are being mapped with Craig's artificial eye implant. They hope that enough auditory information can someday be sent, through implanted electrodes, to allow patients to understand speech.

Because auditory cortex stimulation is more difficult, development of a usable artificial ear will take a long time. If it's successful, however, it will help the many deaf persons who have suffered damage to the auditory nerves. Only auditory cortex stimulation will allow them to hear again.

CHAPTER 4...
THE ARTIFICIAL HEART

IF YOU WERE TO THINK OF YOURSELF AS AN INDUSTRIAL COR-poration, your brain would be the manager and your heart the labor leader. Your brain decides, consciously or unconsciously, what has to be done, and your heart provides the work to keep all departments functioning. Without your brain to send the signals, the industry would fail for lack of leadership; without your heart to keep all systems going, the work would grind to a halt.

When labor and management get together to negotiate about wages, each side brings its own statistics to the bargaining table. Your heart could present an impressive list of figures:

The heart beats more than one hundred thousand times a day, and rests for only a fraction of a second between beats. If you live a normal lifespan, it will beat a total of 3,200,-000,000 times—that's three billion, two hundred million.

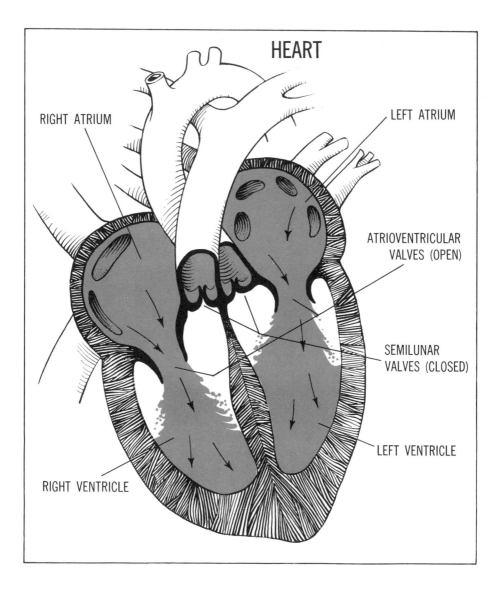

HEART

RIGHT ATRIUM

LEFT ATRIUM

ATRIOVENTRICULAR
VALVES (OPEN)

SEMILUNAR
VALVES (CLOSED)

LEFT VENTRICLE

RIGHT VENTRICLE

The right side of the heart fills with blood which has come to it from all parts of the body except the lungs. The left side fills with blood which has come from the lungs.

When you're sitting still, your heart pushes about 2.25 ounces of blood through your body with each beat. That's 4.7 quarts per minute, or 70 gallons per hour. When you walk at a normal pace, the output doubles. When you play a fast game of tennis, it may quadruple.

Each day, your heart pumps eight to ten tons of blood. In a lifetime, your heart will move two million barrels of blood.

How can an organ no bigger than your clenched fist do such an awesome amount of work?

HOW THE NATURAL HEART WORKS

You think of your heart as one organ beating inside your chest. To understand how the heart works, it might be easier if you would think of two distinct hearts, joined together side by side and pumping at the same time, but each with its own job to do. The right side of the heart sends blood to the lungs, the left side of the heart sends blood to the rest of the body. Each side has two chambers, or hollow areas. The upper chamber is called an atrium, the lower chamber is called a ventricle.

In the right side, the atrium fills with blood which has come to it from all parts of the body except the lungs. This blood— about two ounces of it per beat if you're resting—drains down to the right ventricle. The ventricle then squeezes together in a contraction which pushes blood toward the lungs. This happens about sixty-eight times a minute while you're resting.

On the left side, the atrium fills with blood which has come to it from the lungs. This blood, again a bit more than two ounces of it, drains down to the left ventricle. The left ventricle then contracts to send blood to all parts of the body except the lungs. The left ventricle and the right ventricle contract at the same time, each ejecting the same amount of blood.

When the blood from the right ventricle reaches the lungs, it releases a bit of moisture and a lot of waste gas, mostly carbon dioxide. It picks up oxygen in the lungs, and returns to the left atrium.

When blood leaves the left ventricle, it moves through vessels which divide into smaller and smaller vessels reaching all the body tissues. Then the blood gives up its nutrients and oxygen, and picks up waste liquids and gases. Most of the liquid wastes are filtered out through the kidneys, and the gaseous wastes are carried in the blood to the right atrium and ventricle and from there to the lungs again.

The blood leaves the left ventricle through a single large blood vessel called the aorta. The aorta divides into arteries, which divide into arterioles, which divide into capillaries, some of which are so narrow that blood cells have to line up in single file to pass through them. This arterial network carries blood away from the heart.

The tiny capillaries then come together into venules, which come together into veins. These combine into the two large veins, the inferior vena cava and the superior vena cava, which return blood to the right atrium of the heart. The venous network carries blood back to the heart.

All the blood pumped by the right side flows through the lungs. In contrast, the blood pumped by the left side is spread through all the organs and tissues of the body except the lungs.

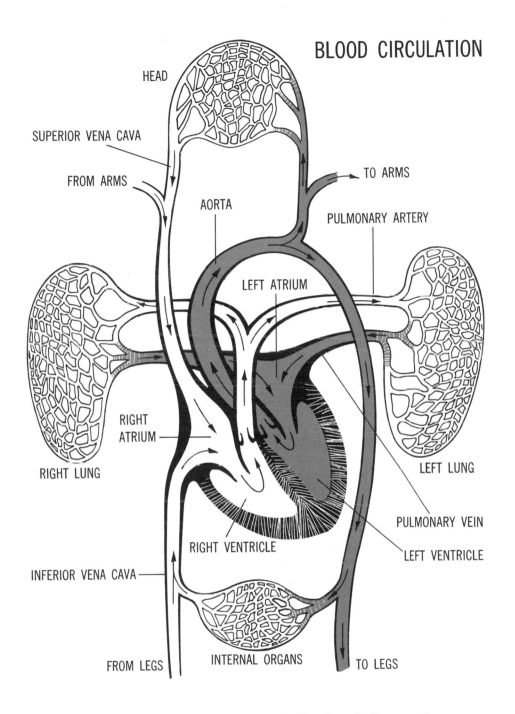

BLOOD CIRCULATION

HEAD

SUPERIOR VENA CAVA

FROM ARMS

TO ARMS

AORTA

PULMONARY ARTERY

LEFT ATRIUM

RIGHT ATRIUM

RIGHT LUNG

LEFT LUNG

PULMONARY VEIN

RIGHT VENTRICLE

LEFT VENTRICLE

INFERIOR VENA CAVA

FROM LEGS

INTERNAL ORGANS

TO LEGS

When the right heart contracts, it sends blood to the lungs to be oxygenated. The left heart contracts to send oxygen-rich blood to all parts of the body. The arterial network carries blood away from the heart; the venous network carries blood back to the heart.

Your blood leaves your left ventricle, flows through your body, and comes back to your right atrium. Then it leaves your right ventricle, flows to the lungs, and comes back to your left atrium. All the time the blood is flowing in only one direction. In order to keep the blood moving always in the same direction, the heart and blood vessels are equipped with valves which close to prevent blood from flowing backward.

The valves between the upper and lower chambers of the heart are called atrioventricular valves, or AV valves. They open downward while the ventricles are filling. The atria (plural of atrium) don't have to push very hard when they contract, because 70 percent of the blood has already flowed downward into the ventricles before atrial contraction.

When the ventricles squeeze together to force blood out of the heart, the AV valves must close so that no blood can be pressed backward into the atria. These valves don't close by their own power—they're pushed into a closed position by blood squeezed against them by the closing ventricles.

Once the blood has been pushed into the aorta and the pulmonary artery by contracting ventricles, it must not be allowed to flow backward again when the ventricles relax. Other valves, called the semilunar valves, close at the mouths of the great vessels to prevent this backflow. These valves have little cups (on the side away from the ventricles) which fill with blood to make them close.

Listen to someone's heartbeat. You can do this by putting your ear against the person's chest, or by using the cardboard tube from a roll of paper towels as a stethoscope. You'll hear two sounds with each heartbeat, sounds which doctors and medical students describe as "lub dub." The first sound, the "lub," is lower pitched and a bit softer. That's the sound of the AV valves closing when the ventricles contract. The second sound, the "dub," is higher pitched and louder. That's the sound of the semilunar valves snapping shut when the ventricles relax.

ARTIFICIAL HEART VALVES

Rheumatic fever is a disease which usually occurs in children, but whose effects are lifelong. When rheumatic fever causes inflammation of the heart valves, scar tissue may form and fuse together the edges of the valves so that they can't open far enough to allow a sufficient amount of blood through. Or, the leaflets of the valves may become deformed by scar tissue so that they can't close properly.

In 1958, for the first time, a damaged heart valve was removed from a patient, and replaced with an artificial man-made valve. Since that time, thousands of lives have been saved by implanted artificial heart valves.

There are many kinds of artificial valves made of many different materials—Dacron, Teflon, Silastic rubber, titanium, stainless steel, and combinations of these materials. None of the valves are perfect. Because they're made of man-made materials which don't work exactly right, mechanically or chemically, inside the human body, the artificial valves may cause certain problems. One of the biggest problems is the formation of blood clots on the man-made materials. Some patients with artificial heart valves must take medicines every day to keep their blood from clotting normally. Nevertheless, it's better to have a not-quite-perfect artificial valve than a severely damaged natural valve.

Until very recently the most widely used artificial heart valve has been the Starr-Edwards "ball-in-a-cage." This valve looks like a bird cage with only three or four spokes. Inside the cage is a ball. The bottom of the cage is an open ring a bit smaller in diameter than the ball.

When the Starr-Edwards valve has been placed inside a patient's heart, forward-flowing blood forces the ball to the top of the cage, allowing blood to flow around the wires and the ball. Then, when the blood attempts to backflow, the ball is pushed back against the ring, blocking it and closing the valve.

Today the most successful valve replacements are porcine heterografts—porcine means pig; heterograft means a graft taken from a species other than man. In other words, heart valves taken from pigs are being used to replace damaged valves in people. And they're working very well.

When the heart valves are removed from pigs, they're sewn to a Dacron-covered frame. Then they're sterilized and treated chemically in a process similar to tanning leather. Later the valves are put into quarantine to make certain that no abnormal bacterial growth exists on them. As they're sewn into place in the patient, the stitches are passed through the Dacron frame. Pig valves are superior to valves of man-made materials because they cause less clotting—patients who have had them implanted need to take anticlotting medicine for

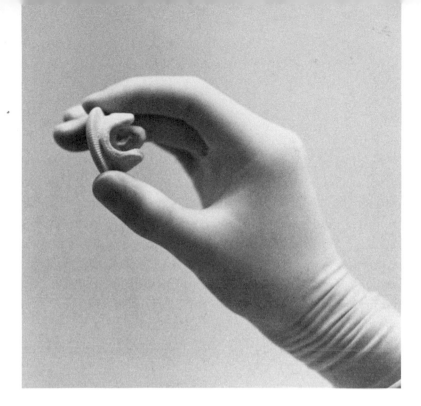

A porcine heterograft—a replacement valve made from the heart valve of a pig.

only six to eight weeks after their operations. Another advantage of the porcine valves is that they have a wider opening, and a flow-through that's not blocked by a ball.

THE PACEMAKER

How does the heart know when to beat? It gets a signal from its pacemaker to begin each and every contraction. The pacemaker is the sinoatrial node, or the SA node, buried in the roof of the right atrium just where the superior vena cava joins the right atrium. It's made of specialized muscle fibers, and is about ½ inch by ¾ inch in size.

To start each heartbeat, the SA node generates an electrical impulse which spreads from muscle fiber to muscle fiber, all through the right and left atria, like waves rippling outward from a stone thrown in a pond. In less than $\frac{1}{10}$ second, the rhythmic impulse travels through the atria and they contract.

Another node, the atrioventricular or AV node, is located near the bottom of the right atrium next to the septum (the septum is the wall dividing the two sides of the heart). When the electrical impulse reaches the AV node, the impulse is delayed for $\frac{1}{10}$ second. This delay gives the atria a chance to contract and fill up the ventricles.

The AV node then sends the signal through bundles of fibers which run downward along the septum and fan out over the inner surfaces of both ventricles. In $\frac{3}{100}$ second, the signal has spread through the ventricles and they contract. At a heart rate of seventy beats per minute, the time between contractions is about $\frac{8}{10}$ second.

The SA and AV nodes aren't the only fibers in the heart which can send signals. Actually, almost every cell in the heart can fire by itself. If live heart cells are placed in a test tube filled with a nutrient solution, and if the cells are separated so that they don't touch one another, each cell will beat at its own rhythm. If two of the cells should touch, they'll begin beating together, at the same rate. The SA node is the heart's pacemaker because it's able to fire signals more rapidly than any other part of the heart.

The heart's electrical signals can be amplified and recorded through electrodes placed on a patient's arms and legs. This recording is called an electrocardiogram.

ARTIFICIAL PACEMAKERS

Sometimes transmission of the electrical impulse through the heart gets blocked at one point or another. When this happens, the atria and ventricles may beat at different rates, or may skip beats, or the heart may beat too rapidly or too slowly. Complete heart block can cause unconsciousness, convulsions, or death.

It was discovered in the 1700s that an electrical stimulus will make any muscle contract. This principle is used for patients who have heart block—their hearts can be stimulated electrically with an artificial pacemaker.

An artificial pacemaker looks like a large pocket watch with a wire running from it. Pacemakers may be implanted in two different ways. In one method, the patient's chest is opened, and two electrode heads are sewn against the heart. Wires from the electrode heads run to the power source of the pacemaker, which is left in place under the skin of the abdomen.

In the most widely used method, an incision is made in the upper chest and into a large vein. A wire (called a catheter electrode) is inserted and pushed through the vein into the inside of the right ventricle, and the pacemaker is left in place under the skin of the chest.

Pacemakers need power sources to generate the electrical signals they send to the heart. Most are battery powered, and the best and newest batteries are made of lithium. These batteries must be replaced about every five years, in a simple operation involving an incision through the patient's skin. In

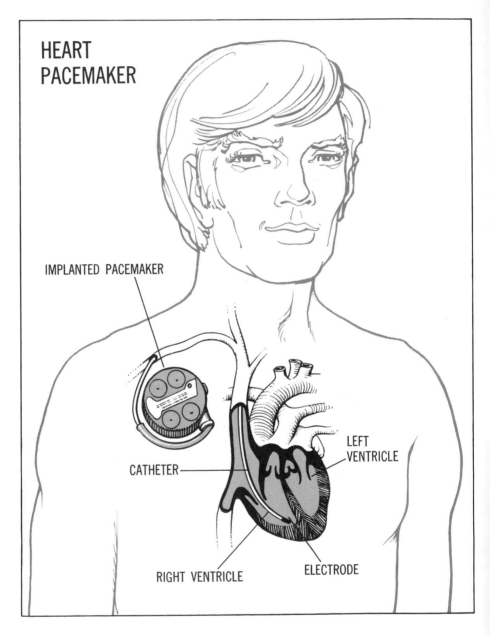

HEART PACEMAKER

IMPLANTED PACEMAKER

CATHETER

LEFT VENTRICLE

RIGHT VENTRICLE

ELECTRODE

In the most widely used method of implanting artificial pace-makers, a catheter electrode is pushed through a large vein and into the right ventricle.

the early 1970s, a nuclear power source for pacemakers was first used. It contains plutonium 238, which generates heat to produce electricity. It can last from five to ten years, and has been implanted in patients both in Europe and in the United States.

The simplest pacemakers cue the heart at a fixed rate of seventy-two beats per minute—they're called fixed pacemakers. Most of the pacemakers in use today are called demand pacemakers. Demand pacemakers have control circuitry which measures the time interval between heartbeats. If the heart is beating normally by itself, they don't fire. If the natural heartbeat becomes too slow, the demand pacemaker then releases pacer pulses to make the heart contract at a normal rate of seventy-two beats per minute.

The artificial pacemaker.

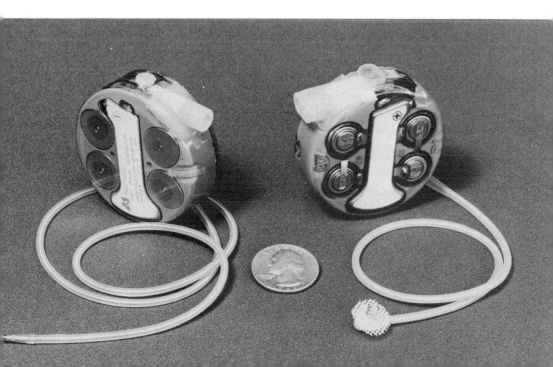

HEART-LUNG MACHINES

Can you imagine a surgeon trying to operate on a beating heart? It would be like threading a needle on a running sewing machine. Of course heart operations must be performed when the heart is stopped; but the heart is a pump which circulates blood, carrying nutrients and oxygen to all parts of the body. When the heart stops, the body's blood supply stops, too. Without a blood supply, muscle and bone can survive for up to an hour, but the brain will begin to be irreversibly damaged in only three minutes.

Since open-heart surgery cannot be performed in only three minutes, a method had to be found which could keep blood flowing to all parts of the body while the heart was stopped. Within the past twenty years, doctors and engineers have developed machinery that can take over the pumping action of the heart for as long as three hours. The procedure is called a bypass, and it's carried out by a heart-lung machine.

During circulatory bypass, blood is taken from the right atrium through a tube, pumped through the heart-lung machine, and returned to the body through an artery in the groin area. In this manner the work of the heart is performed by a machine located outside the body.

The most important part of a heart-lung machine is its oxygenator, which must do the work of the natural lungs—exchanging the carbon dioxide in blood for oxygen. In the natural lungs, tiny air sacs are enclosed in a network of capillaries so fine that they're just wide enough for the red cells to squeeze through. This gives each individual red cell a chance to give up its waste gas and to take on oxygen through the thin membrane of an air sac, an exchange that takes only $\frac{1}{1000}$ second. If the blood-exchange area of both lungs were spread out, it would cover an area of eighty-four square yards, or about a third of a tennis court. There are only two to three ounces of blood in the lung capillaries at any one time—the same amount of blood that the right heart delivers to the lungs with each beat.

An adult, resting, must get rid of two hundred cubic centimeters of carbon dioxide each minute, and must take in two hundred fifty cubic centimeters of oxygen. This rate increases greatly during exercise. You can see that the lungs do an important and complex job, one that is difficult to duplicate in a machine.

Fortunately, the heart-lung machine doesn't have to work as well as the natural lungs do, because when patients are under anesthetic, their body functions are at a minimum. An oxygenator can make do with a gas-exchange area of only seven square yards instead of the eighty-four square yards of the lungs and it can increase efficiency by using 100 percent oxygen instead of the 20 percent oxygen contained in air.

One widely used kind of oxygenator pushes bubbles of oxygen through the blood circulating in the heart-lung machine. This method supplies oxygen to the blood, but it also makes the blood so foamy that it has to be defoamed before it's sent back into the body. When blood is handled a lot in an unnatural way, the red cells become damaged and release hemoglobin which must be cleared away by the kidneys. Also, the protein in the blood gets changed, and very tiny clots may form, keeping the blood from clotting normally. Too much of this kind of damage during surgery causes too great a strain on the body, which is the reason that open-heart surgery can't last longer than three or four hours.

In recent years, researchers have wanted to build a heart-lung machine which would do less damage to the blood. They designed and built an oxygenator in which blood is passed between silicone-rubber membranes that are enveloped in layers of oxygen. The oxygen dissolves into the membranes and diffuses through them into the blood, and the carbon dioxide diffuses out, in a process something like blood dialysis (see Chapter 1). Since blood isn't damaged nearly as much in a membrane oxygenator as it is in a bubble oxygenator, a patient can stay on a heart-lung bypass for much longer periods, as long as several days.

When scientists realized that bypass time could be increased so much, they wondered if they could use membrane oxygenators to help patients with severe lung disease. In clinical trials, they found that the membrane oxygenator can work as an artificial lung, breathing for a patient while his or her own lungs rest and recover.

In July 1976, in Salt Lake City, a young woman named Debbie Anthon developed a bacterial infection after the Caesarean birth of her first child. The infection spread to her lungs and became so serious that she had trouble breathing. As Mrs. Anthon's condition grew more and more critical, her physician, Dr. Alan Morris, suggested that she might be helped by the heart-lung machine.

Debbie's husband Jeff recalls, "Dr. Morris told us that if we were gambling people, the odds were against us. If we did or if we didn't, she had about a 10 percent chance to live, no matter what." Fully informed of the risks of the procedure (no one in that area had ever survived it), the Anthons decided to go ahead with the lung bypass. Debbie was connected to the heart-lung machine.

"It seemed like when she was on the machine she just glowed," Jeff Anthon said afterward. "They had her body covered up, but I could see the machine in operation. I could see that the machine was giving her life."

After three days Debbie Anthon was taken off the artificial lung. Her condition had improved, and continued to improve. Three weeks later she was able to leave the hospital, convinced that the lung bypass had saved her life. Since it's considered to be an experimental procedure, the lung bypass is being tested at eight other research centers on the East and West Coasts.

THE LEFT VENTRICULAR ASSIST DEVICE

The development of the heart-lung machine has allowed operations to be performed today that weren't even thought about twenty years ago. Plastic tubes take the place of diseased arteries. Artificial valves substitute for faulty heart valves. Grafts of vein from a patient's leg are used to bypass clogged coronary arteries. Health experts believe that as many as a hundred thousand open-heart operations are being done each year in the United States.

Sometimes after patients have had heart surgery and have
been on the heart-lung machine for the maximum safe time,
the heart still isn't strong enough to take over the work of
pumping blood. Yet if they were to remain longer on the heart-
lung machine, their blood would suffer the kind of damage
mentioned earlier. They need a device to assist the heart until
it regains enough strength to work on its own, a device which
can give the heart additional time to recover—perhaps a week
or two, or as long as a month.

Scientists at several research centers throughout the country
are developing systems to help out the heart's left ventricle
after surgery. Since the left ventricle is the chamber of the
heart that does the most work, pumping blood to the entire
body, these systems are made to give support to only that part
of the heart. They're called left ventricular assist devices, or
LVADs. After eight years of experimental trials in laboratory
animals (dogs and calves), LVADs were implanted for the
first time in human patients in 1976, at the Texas Heart Institute, by Dr. John Norman.

An LVAD is actually a pump driven by air. The kind of
LVAD implanted in the Texas patients is designed to fit into
the abdomen, for several reasons: the chest is filled with vital
organs—heart, lungs, and great vessels—which can't be easily
pushed aside, while the abdomen holds intestines which can be
moved without too much trouble; an incision in the chest is
more dangerous than an incision in the abdomen, and so
should be avoided whenever possible; and an abdominal implant the size of the LVAD won't interfere with the space the
lungs need to expand in during breathing.

In the LVAD, a flexible tube is inserted into the bottom of the left ventricle, and is attached by a sewn ring. This tube leads downward to a hollow chamber shaped like a small football standing on end. At the top and bottom of the football-shaped pump are two artificial valves—not ball-in-a-cage, but disk valves, which work the same as ball-in-a-cage valves. Inside the chamber walls is a membranous bladder, which fills with blood from the left ventricle. An outside control machine forces air through a tube and into the space between the

Left: *One type of left ventricular assist device (LVAD). Note the ball-in-a-cage heart valve between thumb and forefinger.*

Right: *A left ventricular assist device like this one has been implanted in several patients at the Texas Heart Institute, Houston, Texas.*

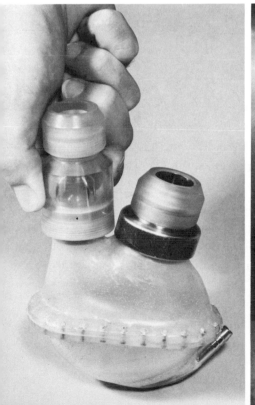 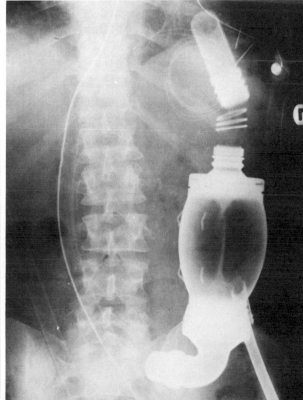

chamber walls and the bladder. The pressure of the air makes the bladder squeeze together, forcing blood out through a tube at the bottom of the pump chamber. This tube carries the blood into the abdominal aorta, where it flows both upward and downward to eventually reach all parts of the body. The air is then pulled out of the pump chamber, allowing it to fill with blood again. All this happens at the same speed as a normal heart rate.

The LVAD can be set to take over all the work of the left ventricle, or only part of it, depending on the condition of the heart. After the patient recovers, the pump must be removed through the original incision in the abdomen. The inflow tube and the outflow tube can be sewn over and left in place.

Even though clinical trials with human patients have taken place, the LVAD is still not perfected enough for general use. But it looks very promising for the future.

THE ARTIFICIAL HEART

In the United States, six hundred thousand people die each year because their hearts wear out, become diseased, go out of control, or are struck with a clot. Perhaps many of these people could go on living if there were some way that they could get new hearts.

In 1967 Dr. Christiaan Barnard of South Africa was able to give a human being a new heart for the first time in history, in the world's first heart-transplant operation. Since then about three hundred forty heart transplants have been performed;

but the patients who have received new hearts have seldom lived for longer than two years afterward. Either their bodies rejected the transplanted hearts; or they had to take so many antirejection drugs that they died from infection; or else their new hearts became diseased, too. Since the additional spans of life gained for these patients have been so brief, fewer and fewer surgeons now feel that heart transplantation is worthwhile. The number of patients living with transplanted hearts grows smaller every year.

Yet the idea of replacing hearts in humans is a good one. The heart is a pump. Why not replace the natural heart with a mechanical pump and let thousands of heart-disease victims go on living? In the very near future, surgeons will probably do just that. Scientists have been working on the problems of heart replacement since 1956.

A total heart replacement, or an artificial heart, is pretty much like a combination of two left ventricular assist devices, but with one very important difference—the LVAD is implanted to help out the natural heart, and when the natural heart recovers the LVAD is removed. In total heart replacement, the natural heart is taken out of the patient's chest, never to be returned. A mechanical heart is implanted which will stay inside its owner for the rest of his or her life.

Considering that scientists have been working on an artificial heart since the mid 1950s, you might wonder why the device isn't ready for use. The biggest problems have been the same ones mentioned earlier—clotting, blood damage, infection, failure of man-made materials to perform well, and difficulty in getting a simple, safe, workable power source. But

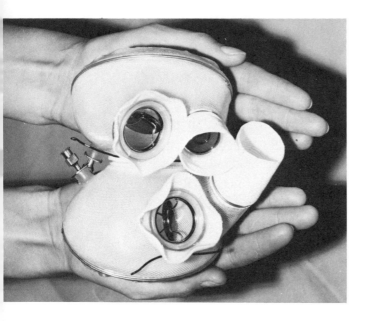

This total replacement artificial heart was developed at the University of Utah.

one at a time, step by step, the problems are being solved. When the first artificial hearts were tried out in calves, the animals lived for only a few hours. Later ones lived for a few days, then weeks, and now for months at a time, as the designs for artificial hearts are continually improved. Animal trials are now so successful that it shouldn't be too long before artificial hearts are ready for clinical trials in people.

An artificial heart was actually implanted in one human patient in 1969. However, so much conflict surrounded the case that it had the effect of slowing down clinical trials from that time till the present.

In the spring of 1969, a forty-seven-year-old man named Haskell Karp came to St. Luke's Episcopal Hospital in Houston, Texas, hoping to get a heart transplant. He was in such critical condition that he was close to death, but no donor organ could be found for him. That is, no person with a healthy heart, who had willed his or her organs for transplantation, and whose tissue matched Haskell Karp's, happened to die around that time.

Karp's doctor, Denton A. Cooley, was convinced that Mr. Karp's life could not be prolonged for many more hours. Dr. Cooley decided to implant an artificial heart in the dying man, in hope that the mechanical heart would keep him alive until a donor heart could be found. The heart was implanted. Mr. Karp woke up, spoke to his wife, and stayed alive for sixty-three hours with an artificial heart pumping blood throughout his body. Then a donor heart was found; and although Haskell Karp finally received a transplant, he died the next day.

Dr. Michael E. DeBakey, who had been instrumental in inventing the mechanical heart which Dr. Cooley implanted in Mr. Karp's chest, was out of the state on the day that the implant took place. He was very angry because he had not been consulted and because he believed that Dr. Cooley should not have implanted a device which was not yet perfected. Dr. Cooley defended himself by saying that without the implant Mr. Karp would surely have died; with it he had some chance, however small.

Mrs. Karp, the patient's widow, sued Dr. Cooley for four million dollars, saying that her husband had been "the unfortunate victim of human experimentation." Even though Mrs. Karp lost the lawsuit, researchers have been very cautious ever since about implanting another artificial heart. They want to be sure that a potential heart implant has been tested enough to be almost foolproof. For this reason researchers keep working to improve their models, implanting them in calves and trying for longer and longer survival records.

Work on total heart replacement is taking place not only in this country, but in other parts of the world—in Berlin, Vienna, Moscow, Rome, and Paris. In the United States, it's being carried out in Salt Lake City, Cleveland, Houston, Boston, and Hershey, Pennsylvania, with the most successful animal experiments occurring in Salt Lake City and in Cleveland.

Each time an artificial heart is implanted in a calf at any of the research centers, the doctors and scientists hope that the animal will live longer than the ones which preceded it. In fact, a spirit of competition has built up as the record for the number of days calves have lived with an artificial heart shifts back and forth from one center to another. The Cleveland Clinic had a Holstein bull calf which survived for 145 days with a total artificial heart. When it died on May 17, 1976, it had set a world record. Then scientists at the University of Utah implanted an artificial heart in a bull calf called Abebe, named after the long-distance runner from Ethiopia who won the Marathon race in the Olympics of 1960 and 1964. When the calf died on May 13, 1977, he'd set a new world record for survival with an artificial heart—184 days.

Both these record-setting calves died not because their artificial hearts failed, but because they'd outgrown them. The Cleveland Clinic's Holstein calf weighed 215 pounds when his artificial heart was first implanted. By the time he'd grown to 425 pounds, his artificial heart just couldn't keep up with the demands made on it by his twice-as-large body.

When the calf Abebe began to grow weaker, indicating that he'd become too big for his artificial heart, University of Utah scientists decided to remove the outgrown heart and implant

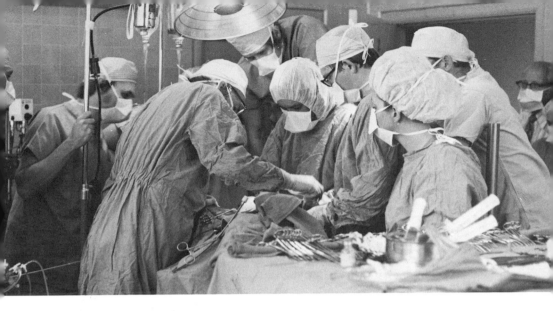

Above: A *team of scientists implants a total artificial heart in a calf.*

Below: A *Holstein bull calf with an air-driven artificial heart exercises on a treadmill.*

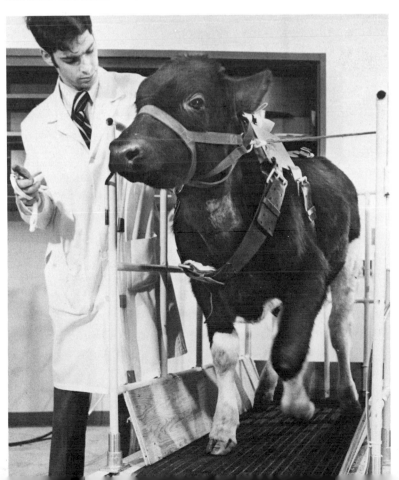

another. But Abebe had a tear in his aorta which the surgeons weren't able to repair, so the follow-up replacement heart couldn't be sewn into place.

In an operation to give a calf an artificial heart, the calf's chest is opened and its circulation is taken over by a heart-lung machine. At the University of Utah, most of the natural heart is removed, but about half of the atria is retained, including the aortic and pulmonary artery valves. At other research centers, the whole heart is removed, including all four valves. Then the artificial heart is sewn into place. Total pumping of both sides of the artificial heart is begun, and the heart-lung machine is stopped. A chest drainage tube is placed in the chest cavity, and the chest is sewn closed, layer by layer. Total operating time—five or six hours.

Most of the artificial hearts presently being used in animal trials are driven by air pumped between the heart chamber and a flexible diaphragm, as in the left ventricular assist device. The power source for these air-driven pumps is very large—it can range from the size of a suitcase to that of a refrigerator.

Artificial kidney machines are very large, too, but patients have to be connected to them only three or four times a week, for several hours each time. A patient with an artificial heart would need to be connected to its power source constantly, for every minute of his or her life. With a power source the size of a refrigerator, the patient would never be able to move around at all. And in addition to size, air-driven power sources cause problems because of the tubes that extend from the console through a patient's skin and into the body. Organisms can travel along the tubes and cause serious infections, no matter how careful and sanitary everyone tries to be.

Although researchers are using the bulky, air-driven power consoles while they attempt to perfect the heart device itself, they realize that eventually they'll have to invent a much smaller power unit if artificial hearts are ever going to be practical for human patients. Probably the best power source for a total artificial heart will be a battery-operated electric motor. Instead of using pressurized air to force a bladder or diaphragm to expand and contract, an electric motor can push a piston against a diaphragm, first in the left heart and then in the right heart. At the present time, though, batteries which are lightweight, long-lasting, and strong enough just aren't available.

Another potential power source for an artificial heart is nuclear energy. Researchers are working on one design that can use plutonium 238 to generate enough heat to turn a small amount of water into steam. The steam would move a piston to drive the heart, then condense, return to the chamber, and start a new cycle. Another design would use the heat to expand a gas (argon), rather than water/steam.

An atomic-driven heart would be so compact and long-lasting that it could be implanted completely inside the patient, with no outside wires or tubes. But it does have some very serious drawbacks. It creates heat which has to be dispersed somehow, probably in the blood. The heat, which may become as high as 112° Fahrenheit, would be carried into the bloodstream, where it could raise the temperature of the entire body to 99°—tolerable enough.

The biggest worry with a nuclear-powered heart is radiation. Patients would probably lose their fertility, and might develop leukemia. Not only that, close family members could be exposed to the same dangers. And if by some incredible accident the nuclear power pack should break open, the lives of people in an area all around would be in danger.

It seems as though the best bet for an artificial heart power unit will be the electric motor, as soon as engineers come up with the right kind of battery. In the meantime, since the artificial heart has been working so well in experimental tests with calves, it's possible that it may be implanted in a human even before the power problem is solved. If patients have a choice of dying or of being hooked up with six-foot lines to a large, noisy machine, they may well choose the machine.

In years past, many people had to spend their lives inside large iron lungs which they could never leave. Air-driven consoles for artificial hearts may turn out to be less restrictive than iron lungs, if the consoles can be reduced to a size which patients can wheel along in large hospital carts.

How long will it be before an artificial heart is implanted in a human being? Dr. Yukihiko Nosé of the Cleveland Clinic Department of Artificial Organs says that although current animal experiments are encouraging, "We still have to develop a fully self-contained artificial heart. That's still far into the future." Dr. Valery Shumakov, director of the Moscow Institute of Transplantation of Organs and Tissues, believes that a total heart replacement is not likely until after the year 2000, but that within the next three years patients can be placed on artificial hearts until donor hearts for transplants are found for them.

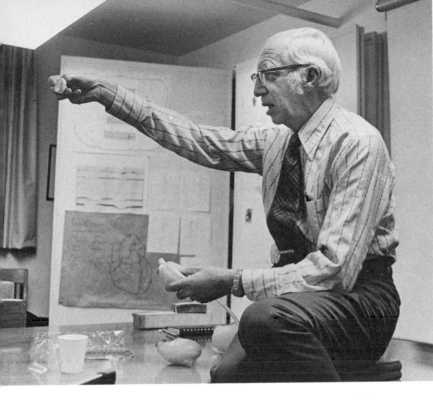

Dr. Willem Kolff demonstrates a model of the artificial heart.

Dr. Willem Kolff, director of the University of Utah's Division of Artificial Organs, always has the same answer when he's asked how soon an artificial heart will be implanted. "I will be very disappointed if the heart is not ready for clinical use in three years," he says, "and three years ago I said the same thing." Dr. Don Olsen at the University of Utah says that an air-driven heart could right now be "implanted in a man's chest and sustain life, perhaps for a year." And Dr. John Lawson, who supervised the care of the calf Abebe, says that when calf trials are 95 percent successful, we'll be ready for clinical trials in humans.

No matter whose opinion you decide to take, it seems certain that artificial hearts will be in use well within your lifetime.

CHAPTER 5...
ARTIFICIAL ARMS AND LEGS

IN AUTUMN OF 1973, EDWARD MOORE KENNEDY, JR., LOST HIS leg. Twelve-year-old Teddy, son of the senator from Massachusetts, had developed a rare form of cancer which affected the cartilage next to the bone in his right leg. His only chance for a cure involved amputation, which was performed as quickly as it could be arranged.

The finest doctors and orthopedic specialists in the country were available to help Teddy Kennedy, to make certain that he would walk again as normally as possible. The procedures they used were relatively new, having been tried for about a decade on a number of amputees, and having been proved effective.

On the operating table, surgeons cut through flesh, then sawed the bone about three inches above the knee. A sufficient amount of skin and tissue was left to be drawn over the bone end to make a good, firm padding. Orthopedic surgeons have come to realize that when a limb is removed, a well-shaped,

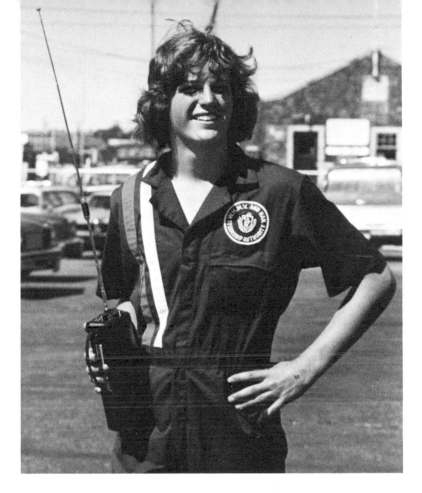

Ted Kennedy, Jr., has recovered from his bout with cancer and is leading a normal, active life.

workable limb termination must be constructed of the remaining tissue. This is the most important part of amputation surgery, because the shape of the limb termination, or stump, is crucial for the proper fitting of an artificial limb.

When surgery was completed, but while Teddy was still on the operating table, a bioengineer covered the wound and the stump with a plaster cast. The cast not only prevented swelling of the damaged flesh, it also was used as a site to attach Ted-

dy's first, temporary artificial leg. The temporary leg, made of
aluminum, was put in place immediately so that when Teddy
woke up he wouldn't experience the shock of seeing an empty
spot in the bed where his leg had once been.

The first day after surgery, he was up and taking steps,
supported by his father. These first steps were painful, but
after a few days he was able to walk up and down the hospital
corridors. Daily sessions in physical therapy helped him learn
to propel the artificial leg, and by the time he left the hospital,
he was able to walk by himself, using crutches.

Four weeks after surgery, the temporary leg was replaced
by a permanent prosthesis. (Prosthesis means any artificial
part which replaces a natural body part. It may be an arm, a
leg, a breast, a hook, and so forth.) Following a procedure
used with all amputees, prosthetics specialists made a cast of
Teddy's limb termination, and later a mold was made from the
cast. In just a few days he had a well-made leg which fit him
perfectly. Four months after the operation Teddy went skiing,
using a specially made pair of skis. Over the next few years he
was able to resume almost all his normal activities, even play-
ing football with his family.

PROSTHETICS CONSTRUCTION

Artificial legs are made in many different ways, depending
on the manufacturer. In one method, a socket of polypropy-
lene plastic is fitted over the mold of the stump. Then a rigid
outer shell is formed around the socket, like a mitten over a

glove. The outer shell is the part of the artificial leg that is seen, and the socket is the part that fits over the stump and holds the leg in place. Like the glove inside a mitten, the socket can be pulled out of the outer shell for any adjustment that needs to be made for proper fit. When young persons wear artificial limbs, both the sockets and the limbs must be adjusted or replaced as the patients grow.

Wearers like their artificial legs to be cosmetic, that is, to look as much as possible like real legs. In one process to make a real-looking below-the-knee prosthesis, the makers rub the patient's remaining natural leg with silicone oil, and pull a cotton stockinette over it. The leg is then coated with liquid silicone rubber, and the coating is repeated. Next a pantyhose is fitted over the leg, and the silicone rubber is allowed to harden. This makes a mold of the natural leg, a mold which can be peeled off like a sock. The mold then has to be turned inside out to match the shape of the opposite, missing limb. (Otherwise the patient would have, say, two right feet.) The structural core of the artificial leg is placed inside the mold, which is then filled with polymer foam. After the foam hardens and the mold is removed, the patient has an artificial leg to match the real leg, one which is wear resistant, has been colored to the correct skin tone, has a natural texture, and is easily cleaned. Above-the-knee prostheses are more complicated because of the knee joint, but this method can be adapted for them.

Sometimes artificial legs are held on with straps or webbing, but the newest ones are held in place by suction. The prosthesis fits so exactly that there's no air space between the stump and the socket, which makes the prosthesis stay on unless the wearer deliberately wiggles out of it. Artificial arms are also attached by the suction method.

USING ARTIFICIAL LIMBS

Artificial legs are easier to operate than are artificial arms. Walking and standing are relatively simple functions, pretty much automatic. Although you are able to rotate (partially) your knee and your ankle, you don't have to do that while you're walking—the knee and ankle move in only one plane as you walk. To keep you upright, your knee must lock when it's bearing your weight during walking and when you're standing still. This locking action can be duplicated rather easily in an artificial leg. Patients usually learn to use their artificial legs in just a few weeks, although it takes them longer to learn to walk without a limp. Generally, the younger the patients, the more easily they adjust to new legs and the more naturally they are able to use them.

Patients are very willing to practice with their artificial legs because they're so anxious to get around again. It's that same desire for mobility and independence which has led to so many devices to help the blind. A patient will put up with a lot of discomfort, and will practice long hours, to be able to move without help from one place to another.

Not so with artificial arms. A person needs two legs to walk with; a person with one good arm, however, is able to do a lot of the things that a two-armed person can do. If an artificial arm is heavy, or uncomfortable, or too complicated to use, the patient may decide that it isn't worth the effort, and choose to get along without one.

Of course, if an arm is essential to the wearer's occupation, he or she will put up with the discomfort of wearing it. Almost five hundred years ago in Germany, a certain knight named Götz von Berlichingen earned his living the way most knights did in those days—by fighting. Götz was no storybook hero in shining armor—he put together a band of knights called free lances (which means that they were willing to work for anyone who paid them), and they burned, pillaged, looted, and raised havoc from one end of the countryside to another. According to German historian David Strauss, "It would be absurd to imagine that those knights drew their swords through an unselfish wish to protect the oppressed. They were not only cruel but avaricious." Götz himself bragged, "I have carried on feuds and taken risks; happiness . . . has been my lot."

In 1505, Gotz's right arm was shot off in battle. Obviously, if a plundering knight lacks a right arm to smite with, he has a major occupational handicap. A few years later, a clever metalworker fashioned an artificial arm for Götz von Berlichingen, who was known ever afterward as the Knight of the Iron Hand.

Götz's prosthesis wasn't just a showpiece; it actually worked. Attached above the elbow with leather straps, the arm had movable jointed fingers, of which the forefinger and thumb could actually be controlled to grasp and loosen. Götz used his good hand to work ratchets and levers in the artificial hand; these opened and closed the finger and thumb, and locked them

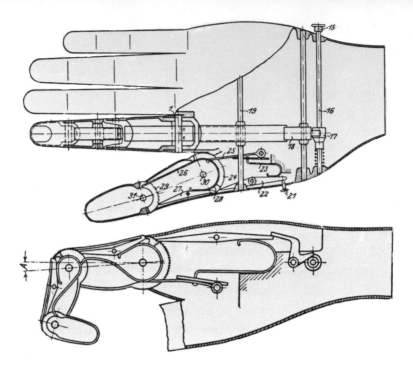

The artificial hand of Götz von Berlichingen could be worked with gears and levers.

into place when Götz wanted to grip something. The three outer, nonmechanized fingers could be bent into a clenched position when they were pressed against a hard surface. Apparently the prosthesis worked very well. It was said that Götz could hit harder with it than he could with his natural arm—a bonus for a man who lived by bashing heads.

Although no one knows for certain, Götz was probably right-handed. When he lost his natural right hand, he used his prosthesis for the heavy-duty work of hitting and smashing; the fine, delicate control functions were taken over by his left hand. In other words, Götz became left-handed. Right or left handedness is something that can be changed if a person loses the use of the predominant hand. Many specialists believe that artificial hands are needed only for the gross (large) functions of holding and grasping, provided the patient still has one good arm.

If a one-armed person works as a machinist, a seamstress, or a carpenter, that person will need two working hands and will be more willing to learn to operate an artificial arm. Mechanically operated arms (those worked by cables and pulleys) require a great deal of concentration. The patient must round a shoulder or twitch a muscle to move the arm, then must bring forward the other shoulder to lock the device in place. All sorts of body movements are necessary to activate the cables and locks, which means that the person must constantly be thinking about arm movements. Only 10 to 15 percent of the patients fitted with these cable-controlled artificial arms actually use them, and only 1 percent get really good at controlling them. Without strong motivation, patients aren't likely to bother with mechanical arms.

THALIDOMIDE CHILDREN

It was once believed that if armless children were fitted with prostheses while they were very young, they'd grow up using their artificial arms in a natural way, without having to concentrate so hard. This theory was tested as a result of a widespread tragedy during the 1960s, when thousands of infants were born without arms, or with only very rudimentary arms. They were called thalidomide children.

In the late 1950s and the beginning of the 1960s, a drug named thalidomide was prescribed as a tranquilizer for a number of women during early pregnancy. These women gave birth to children with various deformities, the most common being missing or deformed arms. Some of the babies had no upper limbs at all, while some had small weak fingers, or hands attached to their shoulders, or rudimentary arms of various lengths.

The children were fitted with prostheses, but because the artificial arms were heavy and awkward and didn't work as well as their own rudimentary hands, most of the children grew discouraged with the prostheses and gave them up. Until very recently, a natural-acting artificial arm just wasn't available.

Persons with birth deformities make up only a very small percentage of the patients who need artificial arms. Most upper-limb prostheses are worn by amputees—patients who have lost their arms because of war wounds, accidents, or disease. Many elderly patients must have limbs amputated because of circulation problems. Artificial arm designers generally concentrate their attention on the problems of amputees.

HOW NATURAL ARMS WORK

Your natural arm can be raised and lowered at the shoulder. It also bends up and down at the elbow and the wrist. It can be rotated at the shoulder, elbow, and wrist, and the fingers can be opened and closed. All these movements can be made in combination, so that you're able to move your arm into any position you wish.

You read in the previous chapter that if your body were a corporation, your brain would be the management and your heart the labor. To carry this analogy farther, in the factory that is your body, your muscles are the skilled craftsmen and your nerves are the messengers which carry instructions to the muscles. This is the way it happens:

Without giving it much thought, you decide to pick up a glass of water sitting on the table. Your brain forms an instant picture of the action you're about to take, and sends commands through nerves that connect to the muscles which will be used in the movement. The nerves fire, causing contractions of the correct muscles in your fingers, wrist, and arm, and you pick up the glass.

As you do, the nerves in your fingers and hand send back the message to your brain that the glass of water feels the way you expected it to feel, that all systems are working normally. If, however, the glass unexpectedly contained boiling water, this information would immediately reach your brain, and you'd drop the glass or at least put it down quickly. And if the substance in the glass didn't turn out to be water, but instead was heavy mercury, your brain would make immediate adjustments so that your muscles would work harder to grip the glass and keep it from falling. This return of information to the brain is called sensory feedback.

Have you ever tried to pick up something when your hand was completely asleep? That will give you a small idea of what it's like to be without sensory feedback. Obviously, artificial arms can't provide sensory feedback to the brain because they don't have nerves. Persons with artificial hands can't tell

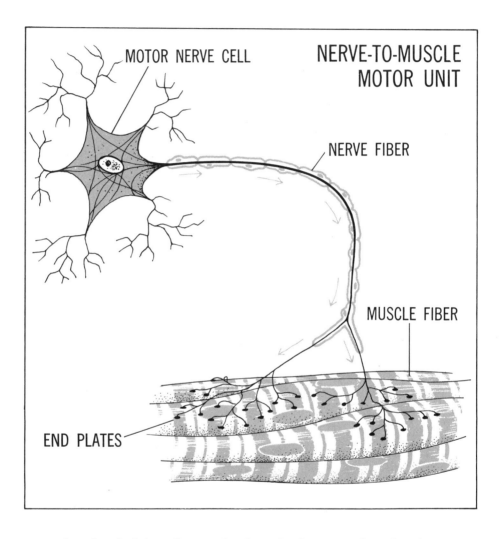

MOTOR NERVE CELL

NERVE-TO-MUSCLE
MOTOR UNIT

NERVE FIBER

MUSCLE FIBER

END PLATES

An electrical impulse speeds through the nerve, branches into nerve fibers and fires muscle cells.

whether an object is hot or cold, heavy or light, or whether they've got a good enough grip to lift it. All the things you can normally tell by touch, persons with artificial arms must tell by sight—they must look to see whether the hand is performing the job it's supposed to be doing. That's one reason why hooks are better than cosmetic hands—they're easier to see around. They take up a lot less space than the more natural-looking artificial fingers.

Every movement your arm makes is controlled by a special set of muscles. Each muscle is made up of thousands or millions of fibers, and each fiber is controlled by an individual nerve ending. (In discussing muscle, the terms "cell" and "fiber" mean the same thing.) Signals which travel from the brain and spinal cord to these nerve endings are actually electrical impulses. As an impulse arrives at the end of a nerve fiber, it releases a tiny amount of a chemical called acetylcholine, or ACh.

This acetylcholine touches off another impulse called the action potential, which causes muscle fiber to contract. Once an action potential has started a contraction, it's an all-or-nothing affair—it can't be stopped or changed in midstream. Each single fiber in a muscle must be fired individually, which is made possible because a single controlling nerve splits up into thousands or millions of nerve fibers, one going to each separate muscle cell. As the electric impulse speeds through the nerve, it branches into the fibers and fires all the muscle cells simultaneously. All this happens in a split second, after which the muscle fiber is ready to contract another time.

THE ARTIFICIAL ARM

Whenever an action potential passes along a muscle fiber, a small portion of the electrical current spreads away from the muscle, as far as the skin. These currents, called electromyographic or EMG signals, can be picked up from the skin by sensitive instruments. EMG signals are the basis for the most exciting concept in artificial arms.

In 1947, research was begun on the use of EMG signals to work artificial arms, but at that time electronic parts were too large and heavy to make the idea practical. During the 1960s, an artificial arm called the Boston/Liberty arm was developed using EMG signals, but problems arose with the interpretation of the signals. Today, aided by the miniaturization of electronic parts and advances in research on muscle signals, scientists at the University of Utah have designed a prosthetic arm which works almost like a real arm. It's activated by EMG signals coming from the muscles of an amputee's arm stump, shoulder, and back.

Dr. Stephen Jacobsen, the researcher most responsible for the development of the Utah arm, demonstrates it in his office in the Merrill Engineering Building on the university campus. He clips a metal clamp, a few inches wide, onto his left forearm, and holds an artificial arm prosthesis in his right hand. A wire runs from the clamp to the prosthesis. As Dr. Jacobsen's left arm moves up and down, the artificial arm moves too, exactly duplicating the motions of Dr. Jacobsen's left arm. Although to the observer the arms seem to be moving at exactly the same split second, the scientist points out that the

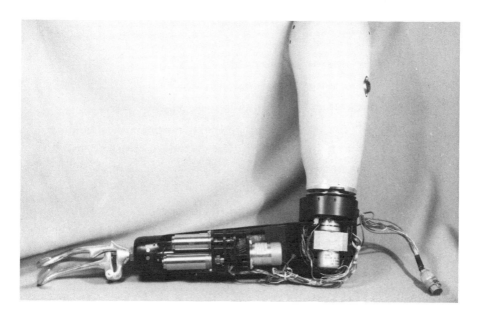

One version of the Utah arm, showing the parts that make it work.

artificial arm movements actually lag by $\frac{1}{50}$ second.

"The Utah arm isn't the first to work on EMG signals," Dr. Jacobsen explains, "but so far it's the best." Externally powered artificial arms must fill certain needs, he points out. In order for them to be accepted by amputees (and what good is an arm if it isn't going to be worn?), an upper-limb prosthesis should be:

> quiet—the motors, batteries, and electronic components which operate the arm shouldn't make much noise
>
> cosmetic—reasonably natural looking
>
> lightweight—the Utah arm, with batteries and components, weighs about two and a half pounds
>
> controllable—the means of making it work should be so

simple and so natural that the patient can learn to
operate it in ten minutes

rugged, fast, strong, and dependable—the arm should be
able to lift weights of five pounds, to react almost in-
stantly, and to work for a reasonable amount of time
before its energy supply needs to be recharged

comfortable—it must not pinch, cut, or catch on clothing

Researchers at other centers have sacrificed some of these
advantages to increase other features—for instance, they've
accepted extra weight to get the benefit of additional electronic parts, or they've accepted more noise to get increased
power. But scientists at the University of Utah believe that
their artificial arm has satisfied all requirements better than
any other prosthesis yet designed. Dr. Jacobsen admits, however, that no prosthesis, now or in the foreseeable future, will
work as well as a natural arm.

The laboratory model of the Utah arm flexes up and down
at the elbow, rotates at the upper arm and at the wrist, and has
a hook which opens and closes. The hook is a special one
designed in this laboratory. It opens wide enough to pick up a
glass. It has interlocking utensil grips, so that it can hold a
knife well enough to cut steak, and can change angles to hold
a spoon or a ballpoint pen. It's able to carry a heavy bucket or
to pick up a single sheet of paper.

Many amputees wear a hook for working, and then change
to an artificial hand for cosmetic reasons (a hand which
weighs a pound by itself). The Utah hook is designed to fit
inside a glove, so that when wearers are concerned about

looks, they can pull the glove over the hook, adding no extra weight. When they want to be functional, they can take off the glove and put it in a pocket.

Just as phosphenes must be mapped for each individual who receives visual cortex stimulation, EMG signals must be mapped for each amputee who uses a prosthetic arm controlled in this manner. That's because size, shape, and muscular development are different in each person, and create different EMG signals. Thanks to computer technology, muscle mapping for the amputee is simple and rapid. The patient sits down in front of a computer with a TV screen. Electrodes are attached to about ten different sites on the back and on the shoulder of the amputated arm, and wires are run from the electrodes to the computer.

The patient is fitted with an upper-arm prosthesis which ends at the elbow, where additional hardware enables it to work a gearshiftlike lever. A dot appears on the TV screen, and the patient is instructed to move the lever, which moves the dot. He or she then tries to get the dot into a little square which has appeared on a continuous curved line on the TV screen. When the patient gets the dot into the box, the computer quickly records the force used and which muscles supplied the force; then the little box moves to another point on the curved line, and the process is repeated.

After about ten minutes, enough information has been gathered about the patient's muscles that the computer can formulate what is called the vector-myogram equation, which is a profile of the patient's set of EMG signals. Then, through microcircuitry, the artificial arm can be programmed to re-

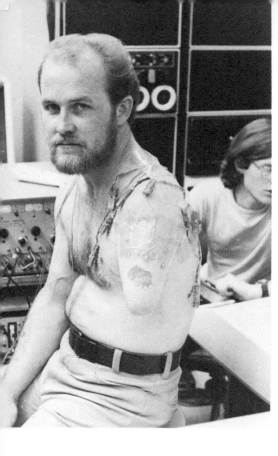
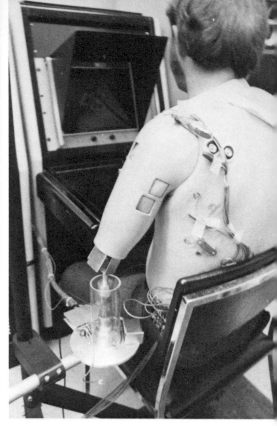
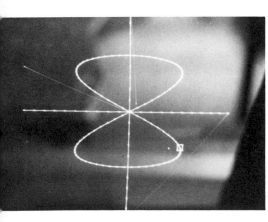
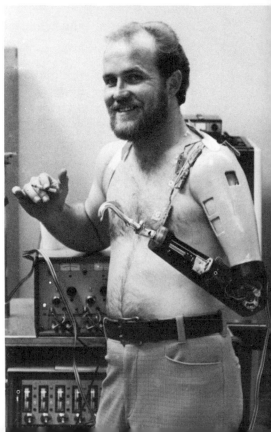

spond to muscle signals in the same way that the real arm would if it were still there. Researchers hope to some day put all the electronic circuits into microcircuit chips, which are paper thin and about ¼ inch square.

In future prostheses, the electrodes which pick up the EMG signals will be molded right into the socket, so that when the amputee puts on the artificial arm, the electrodes will be in the right places to go to work. The present system picks up EMG signals from electrodes attached to the skin of the shoulder, back, and limb termination—about six to nine electrodes. The EMG signals that they pick up are only ⅓ of ¼₀₀₀ of 1 volt. By contrast, overhead fluorescent lights can create voltages inside a person's body of ⁶⁄₁₀ volt—1800 times stronger than EMG signals. Yet the electrodes are able to ignore the stronger voltages inside the body coming from lights directly overhead, and pick up the weaker EMG signals.

When a patient puts on the artificial arm which has been programmed to work on EMG signals, he or she can't activate the arm subconsciously. Although the artificial arm doesn't require the amount of concentration that a mechanical arm

Opposite: *Jack Wiseman lost his arm in Vietnam. In this sequence of photographs, electrodes are taped over chosen muscle sites on his shoulder and back. Wearing a special prosthesis, he works a gearshiftlike lever to try to put the dot into the square on a computer screen. After a ten-minute session, the computer is able to map his muscle signals. The artificial arm is then programmed to work on Jack's EMG signals.*

does, it nevertheless requires some concentration to operate, partly because of the lack of sensory feedback. The patient still has to look at the arm to be certain of its position, and has to think where to move it.

The Utah arm is intended primarily for amputees who have working muscles in their shoulders and arm stumps. But Dr. Jacobsen has encouraging news about thalidomide children, who are now in their late teens. In Great Britain, a researcher named David Cummings Simpson, director of orthopedic bio-engineering at the Princess Margaret Rose Orthopedic Hospital in Edinburgh, is working on prostheses especially designed for thalidomide deformities. Inside the prostheses are buttons which can be controlled by the rudimentary fingers the kids have. Just as a heavy-machinery operator can push levers to control a huge backhoe, these small weak fingers are able to make motions which are duplicated in the much larger prostheses. As Dr. Jacobsen says, "The fingers are primitive, but they get a miraculous sense of the position of the limb. They can outdo anybody, and they can outdo an EMG arm easily."

CHAPTER 6...
BIOMEDICAL MATERIALS

YOU'VE NOW LEARNED A BIT ABOUT BIONIC PARTS FOR PEOple. The devices you've read about aren't terribly complicated, and some of the most creative scientists in the world are devoting their energies to developing these artificial organs. Then why isn't the field farther advanced? Why aren't a lot of people already walking around with artificial eyes, ears, arms, and hearts?

There are several reasons. For one, the scientists are always short of funds to support their research. They spend much of their time writing proposals to ask the government for money —money to buy the special equipment they need for experimenting, to provide laboratories and space to work in, to pay the salaries of bright young assistants who can contribute fresh ideas. Time which scientists must spend begging for money is time spent away from research.

Another factor that delays progress—and perhaps rightly so—is the caution with which artificial organs are tested in the United States. Other countries are more lenient about the safety standards they require for medical experimenting. In the United States, though, the rules are very strict, in order to protect the well-being of patients.

When a new device is invented, it's first tested *in vitro*—that means "in glass," referring to laboratory test tubes and equipment.

Next it is tested *in vivo*, which means "in the body," but always on animals first. The animal trials take a great deal of time. Much data must be gathered before the Food and Drug Administration will allow clinical trials in humans. Even if the animal trials are a complete success, there's no guarantee that the device will work with people.

The first human clinical trials of a new device are permitted on only a few patients at the research center where the device was invented. If these tests are successful, the device may be used on patients outside the center, but only after a great deal more technical and medical data has been collected. Also, during each stage of testing, information is gathered on legal, ethical, and social problems which might arise with use of the device. As an example, before the left ventricular assist device could be implanted in a human patient, the National Heart and Lung Institute called a meeting. Everyone involved in the development of the LVAD was invited to attend, in order to set up guidelines for its first clinical trial. Here are just a few of the questions that were brought up: how will patients be selected? how will consent be given, on what basis, by whom?

what relative quality of life will the patient encounter with the LVAD? what relative quality of dying will the patient encounter with the LVAD? how much will the LVAD cost and who will bear this cost?

After all the safeguards and standards had been established, when the time came for the first LVAD implants, the patients who received them were already so close to death that there was little chance that the LVAD or anything else could save them. It was the same with the first patients who used Dr. Kolff's kidney dialysis machine. The attitude of most doctors has always been, "This patient is about to die. Since nothing else can be done to save his life, perhaps I'll allow the researchers to try out their new device on him. He's so close to death that it can't do him any harm, and there may be a chance that it will do him some good."

The doctors' attitude is quite logical and correct. If it's at all possible for a patient to be cured by a standard and proven treatment, no doctor will take the risk of trying out a new and unproven device. Only after all ordinary methods have failed, and there isn't anything else left to use, will a physician take a chance on an untested technique. And only after experimental devices have proven their worth with "hopeless" terminal patients are they allowed to be used on lower-risk patients.

Although lack of funds and caution in testing are partly to blame for the slow progress in producing artificial organs, the biggest obstacle of all is with the devices themselves: the materials they're made of—the plastics, metals, carbons, and ceramics. Time after time, either the materials cause damage inside the body or the body itself damages the materials.

The very first human replacement parts were made with materials found in nature. More than five thousand years ago, primitive medicine men covered gaping wounds with bark or horsehide, clamped together the edges of cuts with ants' pincers, and used tree stumps to replace missing legs. About twenty-five hundred years ago, a writer from India described sutures (stitches) made of braided horsehair, leather strips, cotton fibers, and animal sinews. In A.D. 1550 gold wire was used for sutures. Three decades later, a physician named Petronius repaired a cleft palate with gold plate, and one named Eustachius did the same thing with silver. By the 1800s, doctors were trying out metal plates to fix broken bones.

In the early part of the twentieth century, certain surgeons attempted to use beef bones, ivory, and wooden rods to repair bones damaged in war. They weren't successful. Then medical knowledge began to expand, and by the middle of the twentieth century, scientists were thinking about much more complicated human replacement parts. By that time, plastics and synthetic rubber had come into wide use, and the scientists assumed that whatever materials they needed would soon be available.

Yet when early devices of synthetic materials were implanted and tested, all sorts of complications developed. For example, some ball-in-a-cage heart valves were made with balls of silicone rubber. A few of the balls absorbed lipids (organic compounds which make up fats), became brittle, and broke into pieces which entered the bloodstream. Very dangerous indeed. Steel plates were used to hold together broken bones, and some of the steel plates fractured. Silicone was implanted in breasts, but it shifted to other parts of the body. In addition to these disasters, there were clotting, blood damage, inflammation, and infection.

Of course, these problems occurred over a number of years, not all at the same time. When a complication developed, researchers tried to figure out just what had gone wrong, and then tried to discover what could be done about it.

The first, most important thing they learned was that no one really knows exactly how the body reacts to outside substances, or how outside substances react in the warm, wet,

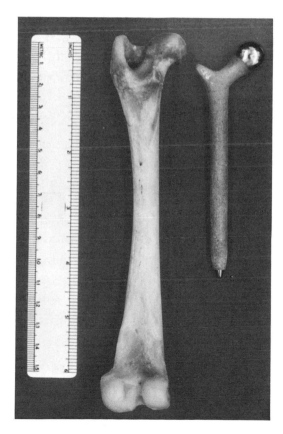

Shown alongside a natural bone is an artificial porous metal bone replacement. The ball-end is polished to a smooth, shiny surface.

sticky, chemical, flowing, moving environment inside the body. A whole new science came into being to answer these questions, the science of biomedical materials, or biomaterials. Beginning in the 1960s, biomedical researchers began to look for and to create new materials specifically designed to work inside human bodies.

They had metals, but no one metal was exactly right for every kind of implant. Metallurgists put together metals in various combinations to search for an alloy which could be shaped easily by molding, casting, or machining and yet would not corrode, deform, crack, or pit in the harsh environment of the body, would not be toxic to the body tissues around it, and would not wear out from the stress put on it by a human body which walks, runs, stretches, and bends. Although a single perfect alloy has not yet been found which can meet all these requirements, there are several very satisfactory metal alloys for implants. Because metals are rigid and rather heavy, they are used mostly to repair broken or damaged bones.

POLYMERS

If you've heard the term "polymer" before, you probably connect it with modern, man-made materials—plastic cups and garbage bags, drip-dry clothes, vinyl furniture. Actually, polymers have been around since the beginning of history. Wool, silk, cotton, rubber, leather, and resins are all natural polymers. It wasn't until the last century that anyone tried to change natural polymers by chemistry.

Back in the 1860s, people liked to play billiards with ivory balls. There was such a demand for ivory that elephant herds in Africa were being wiped out, and ivory came to be in short supply. When a company which manufactured billiard and pool balls offered a prize of $10,000 to anyone who could invent a substitute for ivory, a man named John Wesley Hyatt decided to attack the problem. Hyatt treated cotton with nitric acid to make cellulose nitrates, then added camphor and a solvent to produce a compound which he named Celluloid. Hyatt didn't win the prize for an ivory substitute, but he made a lot of money from Celluloid, which was used for all sorts of things including the high collars which men wore in those days. Unfortunately,Celluloid was flammable.

In 1906, the first completely man-made material arrived on the scene. It was invented by a Belgian-American chemist named Leo Hendrik Baekeland. He mixed phenol and for-maldehyde and added catalysts to form a hard, moldable plastic which was named after him—Bakelite. Baekeland had hit on a workable combination of ingredients strictly by experimentation; neither he nor anyone else understood just what polymers were, or how they acted.

The big breakthrough came in the 1920s when chemists learned to take molecular-weight measurements—the sum of the weights of all the atoms in a molecule. Their findings showed that the man-made materials had very high molecular weights. However, chemists still didn't know what the materials were; they mostly thought that the substances were some highly unusual combinations of matter. Then a German named Herman Staudinger discovered that although the compounds did have very high molecular weights, they were very simple compounds, with long, chainlike constructions. These giant molecules were made by the simple hooking together, or bonding, of atoms into long chains. Staudinger's work led to the development of synthetic rubber, plastics, and artificial fibers, and won him the Nobel Prize in 1953.

When nylon was developed by DuPont in 1935, the rapid growth of the polymer industry began. People started to measure the properties of polymers, and to analyze them. Soon they were tailor-making compounds to fill different needs. By the 1960s the polymer industry—an industry that people hadn't even imagined in the 1920s and 1930s—was turning out more than twenty billion tons of polymers per year. Nylon, Orlon, Teflon, Lucite, Plexiglas, vinyl, styrene, polyester—the list grew longer year after year. Factories made more polyethylene than aluminum. Production of polymers was greater than of any metal except steel. The age of polymers had begun.

Man-made polymers are made from basic chemical raw materials called monomers. A monomer is a single chemical unit. When it reacts with other monomer units to make a chain of repeating units, the result is a giant molecule called a polymer. Hundreds of different monomers can be used to make polymers.

Ordinary organic molecules have rather low molecular weights. The molecular weight of ethanol is 46, of benzene 76, of sucrose 346. The biggest organic molecules have molecular weights which go as high as 1500. By contrast, man-made polymers have considerably higher molecular weights. Nylon's

POLYMER CHAINS

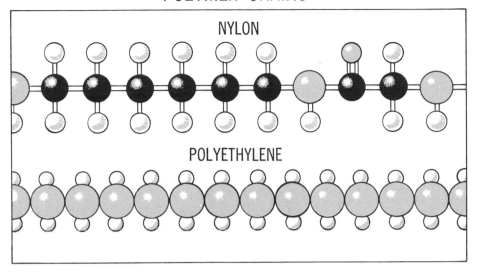

NYLON

POLYETHYLENE

Molecules of synthetic polymer are hooked together to form simple but very long chainlike structures. Some are linear, others are branched or cross-linked.

is about 10,000, Orlon's from 100,000 to 400,000, polyethylene's from about 100,000 into the millions.

If synthetic polymers are made up primarily of carbon, hydrogen, and oxygen, with bits of nitrogen, chlorine, fluorine, silicon, or sulfur, why are their molecular weights so high? It's because the molecules are hooked together to form simple but very long chainlike structures. Some of them are linear—long chains with links side by side like a single-strand necklace. Others are branched—they look like ladders; or cross-linked —they look like the jungle gyms on playgrounds. Linear polymeric materials can be melted or dissolved and can be formed into any shape; the cross-linked ones can't.

These long chains are made of the same or similar molecules, but their lengths vary, even in the same substance. In a polymer, a molecule will repeat itself over and over again, but there's no set number at which it will stop repeating. It may go on and on, building up to an extremely high molecular weight.

Another image will let you see what happens when these giant molecules of polymers are combined with one another. Think of a plate of spaghetti, full of strands of all different lengths. The strands are wound and hooked around one another so that if you put your fork into one end of the mass and move it, the whole mass moves. Polymer molecules—the linear ones, at any rate—combine with each other in just this way.

Researchers test a polymer material which will be used in an artificial heart. The molded diaphragm must withstand millions of flexions.

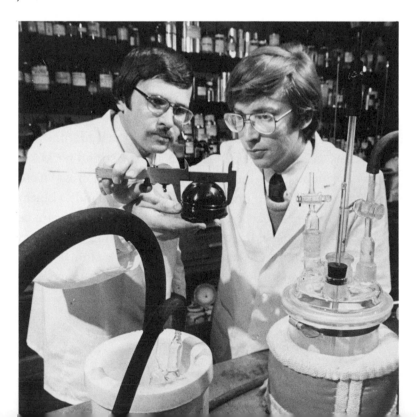

There's a tremendous range in the properties of polymers. Some of them are turned into products that will dissolve in water, and some of them water won't touch. Some are liquid at very low temperatures, yet others won't melt below a heat of 300° Centigrade. Some are elastic—they bend, bounce, and snap—while others are as strong and rigid as steel.

Since polymers can be tailor-made into so many different substances which can do so many different kinds of things, they're the best choice for creating biomedical materials. But the process is not simple—it isn't like dropping in at the chemistry lab to ask the chemist to whip up a batch of polymer with certain characteristics. Even if it *were* that easy to create a new polymer, the scientists wouldn't know, down to the last detail, precisely what to ask for. Not enough has yet been learned about the internal chemistry of the body.

Scientists do know enough to ask the following questions about the polymers they already have, if they're to be used inside the body:

Is it the right polymer for the particular job? Special devices require polymers with special properties.

Is it pure? Any residue from the manufacturing process must be removed.

Can it be shaped into the right form without any change in its properties? Some polymers are so sensitive that the side which was next to the mold acts differently than the side which was away from the mold.

Can it be sterilized without changing its properties? Steam is normally the best way to sterilize implants, but steam melts some polymers and chemically degrades others.

Will the polymer create clots or damage blood? Will it cause inflammation or tissue change? A lot of devices may work fine for a year or two, but what will happen after five years, or twenty? The field of implant surgery is so new that nobody knows what the long-term effects will be.

In spite of these precautions, or perhaps because of them, polymers usually work very well in biomedical implants, from artificial hearts to artificial joints to those oldest implants of all—sutures. And in dozens of implants in between.

CERAMICS

Although ceramics have been mentioned as a biomedical material, along with metals and polymers, their use is still pretty much experimental. Ceramics do have certain properties which researchers consider promising—they don't dissolve in fluid and they won't corrode inside the body. They're particularly good for bone and tooth repair, because bone will bond with a certain kind of ceramic implant.

Also, metals can be coated with ceramics, and ceramics can be combined with polymers. In fact, metals, ceramics, and polymers can all be combined for biomedical implants, to take advantage of the best characteristics of each material. Scientists have learned that in most cases, no one material is best for any implant.

CHAPTER 7...
ARTIFICIAL PARTS FOR PEOPLE

Now for one final, head-to-toe look at bionic parts for people. Devices which have been mentioned in detail in previous parts of this book won't be discussed again, and a few new devices and systems will be mentioned. Here goes—the present and possible future uses of bionic replacement parts:

Plates of metal or of rigid polymer are used to patch holes in the skull caused by war wounds or accidents, particularly motorcycle accidents, which do a great deal of damage to skulls. Metal plates, attached with screws, are also used to hold together fractured bones, mostly the long bones in the legs. These plates must have smooth, rounded corners, be-

BIONIC PARTS FOR PEOPLE

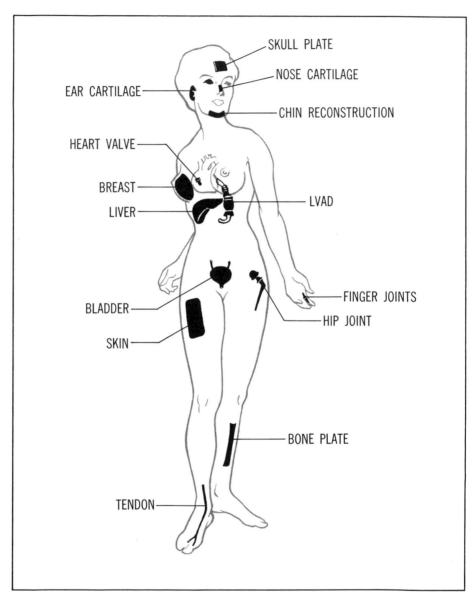

A *number of bionic replacement parts are already in use; others
are being researched and developed.*

BIONIC PARTS FOR PEOPLE

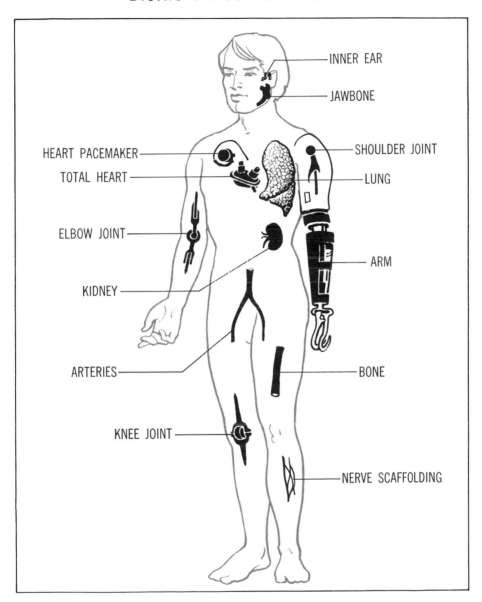

If scientific advancement continues to accelerate, there may come a time when every part of the body can be replaced.

cause sharp, angled corners tend to cause fracturing of the metal. Made mostly of stainless steel, the implanted plates have caused an unexpected modern-day problem. When patients who are patched with plates walk past metal detectors at airport security checkpoints, they ring the buzzer. Imagine explaining to a security guard that you're not really carrying a concealed weapon—it's just the steel plate inside your leg.

Ear cartilage, nose cartilage, chin reconstruction. When parts of the face are deformed because of birth defects, or are damaged in accidents, plastic surgeons can rebuild them with a special high-purity silicone rubber. The reconstruction material is used on the outside of the skin, not inside. It is soft and elastic enough to move and feel like real flesh, but strong enough to stand the stress created when the patient talks, chews, laughs, or sneezes.

The *brain pacemaker* is very new and is still very much experimental. Developed at Tulane University in Louisiana, it's a device consisting of three to five metal electrodes which are placed on the surface of the brain under the back of the skull. Used to relieve the suffering of mental patients, the brain pacemaker sends a small current into areas of the brain associated with pleasant feelings. Although the current can't be felt by patients, the pacemaker's inventor, Dr. Robert Heath, says that it decreases the unhappy and angry feelings associated with psychosis. In its first very limited testings, the brain pacemaker has helped schizophrenic, neurotic, and violent patients.

Bone *joints* can deteriorate because of injury or disease, particularly rheumatoid arthritis and osteoarthritis. The first *total hip replacement* with a metal joint was performed in 1946, but by the 1960s the operation had become almost commonplace. About fifteen thousand total hips are implanted each year in the United States.

When both parts of the hip (ball and socket) were replaced with parts made of the same metal, problems arose, because metal rubbing against metal creates friction. When two different metals were used, they reacted with each other electrochemically. Most widely used today is a combination of metal with polymer—stainless steel for the ball-and-stem, ultrahigh-molecular-weight polyethylene for the socket. Paste made of acrylic plastic is used to attach the socket to bone, and to hold the stem inside the thigh bone.

Stainless steel, of which the ball-and-stem replacement parts are made, is much more rigid than natural bone. At the University of Wisconsin, materials engineers are experimenting with replacement bones made from metal powder. They'll be more similar to natural bone—strong, resiliant, porous, and lighter-weight than solid metal. The ball-ends of the bone implants will be polished to a smooth surface, but the stem parts will be left porous, so that natural bone can grow into the implant and keep it tightly in place. These porous bones have been tested in rabbits and dogs. (See illustration on page 115.)

Two doctors and a biomedical engineer at the University of Michigan have developed a *total knee replacement*. Made of metal alloy, it bends three ways, just like a real knee does. The operation to implant it takes only an hour, and the patient recovers quickly, but as yet the artificial knee is not as strong as a natural knee joint.

Researchers at the University of Arizona have implanted an
artificial wrist in a number of patients. Cemented on one end
to the radius of the forearm, and at the other end to the
metacarpal bones of the second and third fingers, the device
allows nearly normal wrist motions. Its developers believe that
the replacement wrist will probably be as durable as the bones
to which it's attached.

Patients whose hands are crippled from arthritis can have
their *finger joints* replaced. Some finger joints have been made
with hinges, but now most of them are of flexible silicone
rubber, without separate hinges. Patients who have had these
implants have been able to play the piano and type within
weeks after the operation, moving their fingers freely for the
first time in years. Silastic joints are also being used to replace
shoulders and elbows.

Artificial *tendons* are being tested at the United States
Army Institute of Surgical Research. Made of a Silastic sheath
covering a core of Dacron tape, the tendons are being tested
in—of all things—chickens. The chicken was chosen as the
experimental animal because the anatomy of its toe is similar
to that of the human finger; it is prehensile, which means that
it can grasp.

When natural *blood vessels* get clogged with fatty substances from the blood, the largest arteries can be replaced
with tubing made from woven or knitted Teflon or Dacron.
After a while, the replacement vessels become coated with
fibrous protein tissue deposited by the blood, which is good:
the smooth lining discourages clots. Large Dacron replacement vessels can last as long as fifteen years.

These woven artificial blood vessels work very well, when they're wide enough in diameter. However, when they're narrower than six millimeters (about ¼ inch), they can become blocked with clotted blood. At the University of Utah, a research team headed by Dr. Donald Lyman has developed a new polymer which looks very promising for small-diameter blood vessels. "We felt that the problem [of clotting] arose from the mismatch in flexibility between the polymer and the natural vessel," Dr. Lyman explained. "This apparently caused enough trauma at the suture site, as the vessels pulsed, to cause mechanical damage . . . and to initiate clotting." The new polymer, a flexible copolyurethane, allows the replacement blood vessel to pulsate with the natural blood vessel to which it's attached, as blood flows through them. Small-diameter grafts, when they're perfected, will replace damaged arteries in the lower leg, kidney, liver, or brain.

Only the very earliest research has as yet been done on the *artificial liver*. At The New York Blood Center, Dr. Carl Wolf has grown rat-liver tumor cells on hollow fibers like the ones used in kidney dialysis machines. The cells grow on the outside of the fiber membrane, and can metabolize bilirubin, which is one of several functions of the natural liver.

Why are tumor cells used? Because natural liver cells, although they have the ability to regenerate (regrow themselves) inside the body, can't yet be grown as readily in tissue cultures. However, almost any tumor cell can be grown in a tissue culture.

According to Dr. Wolf, "The main use of the artificial liver will probably be to tide someone over an acute period of liver dysfunction until the liver cells regenerate." If it's ever perfected, the artificial liver will be expensive, because instead of being manufactured, it must be grown in a laboratory. At Harvard Medical School, the same principle was used to develop an *artificial pancreas*. Dr. William Chick found that rat pancreatic beta cells cultured on hollow fiber bundles responded to increased amounts of glucose by releasing increased amounts of insulin.

The *bladder*, like the liver, can regenerate itself to a large extent. At the Cleveland Clinic, researchers are working to obtain a material which can be used to reconstruct a damaged bladder, and which will then dissolve as the natural bladder regenerates around it. They took pericardium (the membranous sac which encloses the heart) from cows, treated it chemically, and used it to replace part of the bladder wall in laboratory dogs. When the dogs were sacrificed and examined weeks or months after the implants, researchers found that the artificial bladder had, indeed, supported regrowth of the natural bladder, and then dissolved and disappeared. The method was then tested with five human patients, and in follow-up examinations over the next year, all five patients seemed to be doing well.

Skin, as a grade-school scientist once said, "Holds in what has to stay in, and keeps out what ought to stay out." When large areas of skin are destroyed, as with severe burns, the body is exposed to serious outside infection and at the same time loses heat, fluids, and body nutrients. Skin from cadavers can be used to cover the burned areas until the patient's own skin begins to grow again, or pigskin can be used. Eventually these grafts are sloughed off because of rejection, but by that time the patient may have recovered enough so that skin grafts from other parts of his or her own body can be used to repair the burned areas.

The Naval Medical Research Institute is experimenting with a plastic material which would serve as a replacement for the superficial layer of skin lost through injury or burns. The work isn't very far along, and to date the material hasn't been tested in humans. The U.S. Army is also working on polymeric burn dressings.

Physicians and engineers at Harvard and Massachusetts Institute of Technology have bonded carbohydrates and protein collagen to form a fiber-reinforced material. In animal tests, the material seems promising as a skin substitute for burn victims.

Artificial blood. At the Harvard University School of Public Health in Boston, researchers successfully replaced all the blood of living rats with protein-free artificial preparations. The rats survived, quickly regenerated blood cells and proteins, and continued to grow normally. Because of the complexity of whole blood, no simple artificial mixture can provide all the properties and functions of normal blood; but artificial blood will probably be good enough to sustain a patient during surgeries where such massive blood transfusions are needed that enough whole blood is hard to find.

The most promising artificial blood research uses liquid fluorocarbons—chemical combinations of fluorine and carbon. These compounds can absorb and carry oxygen and carbon dioxide very much the way natural blood does.

THE FUTURE OF REPLACEMENT PARTS

The list of artificial parts for people mentioned here and in previous chapters will have given you some idea of the spare parts now available, and of those which will soon be available.

But what about the far-distant future? Most artificial organs researchers admit that the field is so new that its future possibilities are hard to imagine. If scientific advancement continues to accelerate, there may come a time when every part of the body can be replaced, when no one will ever have to wear out, when humans can become immortal, at least in theory.

The legal and ethical problems surrounding this kind of immortality are just as complex as the technical problems. What about the overcrowding of our planet, if people are routinely patched up to keep on living as new generations arrive on the scene? What about religious beliefs—that there is a time to be born and a time to die? How can there be an afterlife if no one ever dies?

More practically, what nation's economy can afford the tremendous cost of replacing worn-out or diseased parts in every citizen? And if the costs are too immense to allow each citizen to be indefinitely repaired, who will decide which portion of the population is to be kept alive?

"Quality of life" is a term in use even today in the field of artificial organs. Physicians and surgeons must decide in advance whether a biomedical implant is worth the cost and effort—whether the prolonged life that results will be worth living. In the future, if people can be kept alive until they are well over a hundred years old, will they enjoy living or will they merely stagnate in loneliness and misery? If a nation's economic resources are spent to keep its citizens living well past the Biblical three score and ten years, will the nation have enough money left over to pay for education, housing, defense, space exploration, and environmental research? What are the priorities?

The necessary technology is already with us. Barring worldwide disaster, it will increase and expand indefinitely. But the moral and ethical questions have not yet begun to be answered. Perhaps you'd better start to think about them.

CHAPTER 8...
THE CREATORS

RESEARCHERS WHO ARE DEVELOPING BIONIC PARTS FOR PEO-
ple believe that their careers yield a great deal of excitement
and satisfaction. They devote long hours to discovering new
approaches to problems, to laboratory experiments, and to
teaching the young graduate students who are anxious to enter
the field. They come from a variety of educational back-
grounds—in medicine, chemistry, various branches of engineering, in veterinary science, computer science, and others.
The following biographical sketches will acquaint you with
some of the foremost researchers, and with the feelings they
have about their work.

WILLEM JOHAN KOLFF, M.D., PH.D.

Dr. Kolff was born in the Netherlands on February 14, 1911, the son and grandson of a doctor. During his boyhood he had no wish to enter medicine, because he didn't feel that he "could bear to watch people die." But the attraction was strong, and in 1938 he graduated from the University of Leyden Medical School.

In 1950, Dr. Kolff moved to the United States to work at the Cleveland Clinic, becoming a U.S. citizen six years later. He built improved versions of the artificial kidney, designed artificial hearts and blood oxygenators, and developed techniques for preserving organs during transplant operations.

In 1967 he transferred to the University of Utah as head of the Division of Artificial Organs, where he practices as much engineering as medicine. Dr. Kolff says, "I know that some people feel that you can make a biomedical engineer by first letting him study medicine and then engineering. I want to do it another way. I want to have brilliant, young, aggressive people, train them basically, and give them a degree in one of the disciplines. By contacting others, and by their interests and studies in a specified direction, they will learn enough to do what they want to do." Dr. Kolff feels that too much formal training destroys the creative ability of a good engineer— emphasis is too often on analysis rather than creativity.

Though he does not teach regular classes, Dr. Kolff is always willing to lecture when he's asked, delivering the lectures without notes. His son Jack is also a doctor, making the fourth generation of Kolffs to enter medicine.

WILLIAM S. PIERCE, M.D.,
PROFESSOR OF SURGERY

Dr. Pierce relates his background in his own words:

"I have always had a strong interest in mechanical devices and in engineering problems. In my youth I enjoyed learning how things worked, and did a good deal of woodworking. In 1954 I obtained a degree in Chemical Engineering from Lehigh University, and during my senior year, I became interested in the dynamics of blood flow. At about that time I became quite interested in medicine and decided to attend medical school. Soon after my arrival I began studying under a surgeon who had considerable interest in the heart-lung machine and in artificial heart valves (Dr. Charles K. Kirby) and I told him of my idea of using a mechanical pump to replace the heart. Dr. Kirby and I embarked on a research program, and our first publication in the field was in 1962.

"After graduating from medical school at the University of Pennsylvania, I completed cardiothoracic surgical training and spent two years with the National Heart, Lung, and Blood Institute in Bethesda, Maryland.

"At the present time I am Professor of Surgery at the College of Medicine of the Pennsylvania State University, and spend half of my time carrying out a wide variety of operations ranging from cardiac operations in newborn infants to combined coronary artery bypass grafting and valve replacement in adults. I head a group of about twenty-five persons who are involved in the development of the left ventricular assist pump and the total artificial heart. Most all of the time, we have a calf with an artificial heart here at the Milton S. Hershey Medical Center."

DONALD J. LYMAN, PH.D.

Dr. Lyman received his Ph.D. in chemistry at the University of Delaware in 1952. For several years he worked in industry, for the DuPont Company. He then transferred his considerable talents to research at the university level, first at Stanford Research Institute and later at the University of Utah, where he is presently a professor of Materials Science and Engineering, professor of Bioengineering, and research associate professor of Surgery.

Dr. Lyman states, "The past two decades have seen a tremendous increase in the use of biomedical materials in medicine. Although nonbiological materials such as metals have been in use for hundreds of years, the more recent developments have been closely aligned with the development of polymers. The skill and imagination of the surgeon have led to a wide variety of uses. While progress has been made in these areas, there have also been failures resulting from improper choice of materials or usages. Such failures are intolerable and are often avoidable if one has a proper knowledge of the materials available for biomedical uses."

Dr. Lyman predicts, "The future of polymer implants, in at least some cases, concerns implants that will immediately provide a functioning system, yet become a scaffolding on which controlled regeneration of the natural part can take place.

Our major limitation in implant research is the imagination of the investigator," he says. "This imagination, however, must be backed by a solid base of scientific understanding."

Through the efforts of Don Lyman, the nation's first center devoted solely to biomedical polymer research will be established at the University of Utah.

WILLIAM F. HOUSE, M.D.

Dr. William House is president of the Walt Disney Rehabilitation Center, and director of the Cochlear Implant Project of the Ear Research Institute in Los Angeles, California. He received his M.D. degree at the University of California in 1952.

During the early 1960s, Dr. House began to devote his efforts to research on the cochlear implant. "The disappointment and slow progress of the early years have only been overcome by dogged determination to see the thing through," he says. "If it had not been for the encouragement and stimulation from the deaf patients who are the center of the project, it would have died long ago."

Dr. House gives a great deal of credit to Jack Urban, an electrical engineer who had previously developed many optical and television systems for surgical procedures. "Over the years Jack devoted untold hours to the work without financial compensation. The project has now acquired a dedicated staff. None of [our progress] would have happened if this were 'just a job' to them."

STEPHEN JACOBSEN, PH.D.

In second grade (both years of it), they told him to write on the lines, but somehow his letters kept wiggling all over the page. In third grade, they wanted him to memorize the multiplication tables, but the answers continued to elude him. He did not exactly fit into their ways of teaching, and on into his twenties he was not especially fond of school. But Steve Jacobsen did want to be an engineer.

In 1960, after one hundred thirty hours of a D average at the University of Utah, he was notified by the dean's office that, if he wanted to remain in school, he would have to attend at night. After one term in night school, he convinced the department chairman to let him back in as a regular student on the guarantee that he would get nothing below a B. He kept his promise.

Today Dr. Jacobsen is recognized nationally as director of the University's Project and Design Laboratory. "I'm convinced it takes many people to develop a good idea," he says. "I believe in group design. You get the best results out of creative people who see needs and sacrifice individual ego for a good result."

Dr. Jacobsen works seventy or eighty hours a week. The first three weeks of each college term are devoted to convincing his students that "engineers are artists," creative and curious as well as analytical.

DENTON A. COOLEY, M.D.

Dr. Cooley was born in Houston, Texas, in 1920 and was graduated from Johns Hopkins University Medical School in 1944. Filling an internship under Dr. Alfred Blaylock, the young Dr. Cooley was able to assist at the first "blue baby" operation. After military service and further surgical training, he returned to Houston as instructor in surgery at Baylor University, under the chairmanship of Dr. Michael E. DeBakey. Together, they advanced a technique to repair aneurysms of the aorta, and later, at the Texas Heart Institute, Dr. Cooley designed several artificial heart valves. He performed heart transplants in nine patients, but found the rejection problems too great to combat.

In May of 1969, with his associate, Dr. Domingo Liotta, Dr. Cooley performed the first implantation of an artificial heart in a human patient. He is now surgeon-in-chief of the Texas Heart Institute.

JOHN C. NORMAN, M.D.

Dr. Norman was born in Charleston, West Virginia, but went to Harvard to earn his B.A. (magna cum laude) and his M.D. After further studies in Birmingham, England, and at Ann Arbor, Michigan, he joined the staff at Boston City Hospital as an associate professor of surgery. While at Boston, he coordinated a complex research project on the use of porcine (pig) liver perfusion in the treatment of liver failure in man.

He also did extensive research in transplantation of the spleen for hemophilia victims.

In 1972, his work with the abdominal left ventricular assist device led him to the Texas Heart Institute, where the device is now undergoing clinical trials. He's also investigating power sources and materials for use in an artificial heart being tested in calves at the Institute.

JOSEPH ANDRADE, PH.D.

Dr. Andrade earned his Ph.D. in Metallurgy and Materials Science at the University of Denver in 1969. Now at the University of Utah, he holds joint appointments in Materials Science, in Applied Pharmacology, and in Surgery. He's in charge of a group whose task is to develop and test biocompatible materials and he has worked on an artificial flexor tendon for the hand as well as on enzyme electrodes for the testing of biochemicals.

"Research in the field of biomaterials involves studying problems which are truly multidisciplinary," Dr. Andrade believes, "and which involve a large number of variables, only a few of which can be studied at any one time. All of the others must be carefully controlled. People in the field should have the ability to utilize concepts involving many variables. I particularly like the quote by Albert Szent-Györgyi [who won the Nobel Prize in 1937], 'Research is to see what others have seen, and to think what no one else has thought.' "

YUKIHIKO NOSÉ, M.D., PH.D.

Dr. Nosé began work at the Cleveland Clinic Foundation in 1964 under Willem Kolff, who was head of the laboratory at that time. Since 1971 Dr. Nosé has headed the Department of Artificial Organs at the Cleveland Clinic.

A native of Hokkaido, Japan, Dr. Nosé received his M.D. and his Ph.D. degree in surgery at the university there. As one of the requirements for his degree, he attended courses at the University of Tokyo, where he was introduced to the field of cardiac prosthesis research. At that time, he designed a micromotor pump for ventricular bypasses which was implanted in dogs, the first experiment of this kind performed in Japan.

Since 1958 Dr. Nosé has been involved in the development of artificial organs, and he has published papers on the artificial heart, kidney, liver, lung, and bladder, and on oxygenators. He has also contributed to the development of polymeric materials.

Dr. Nosé says, "When I began working on artificial organs, hemodialysis was still risky. I remember the first series of kidney dialyses—60 percent of the patients died. Heart treatment was also risky—a perfusion of ten to fifteen minutes was all we could do.

"Even now the era of artificial organs is just beginning, and we don't know how far we can go. It's a field so complex and sophisticated that it must be accomplished by teamwork—the best surgeons, engineers, polymer scientists and chemists must get together and establish first-class research. Artificial organs is one of the most exciting, challenging fields of the future for anybody interested in medicine or engineering."

INDEX

Asterisk (*) indicates photograph or drawing